T0332480

THE HYPERLIPIDAEMIA HANDBOOK

THE HYPERLIPIDAEMIA HANDBOOK

Dr Martin Godfrey
General Practitioner, Beckenham, Kent, UK
Group Medical Editor on GP *and* Mims Magazine

with a Foreword by
J Shepherd
Professor of Pathological Biochemistry, Royal Infirmary, Glasgow

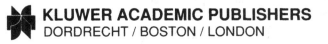
KLUWER ACADEMIC PUBLISHERS
DORDRECHT / BOSTON / LONDON

Distributors

for the United States and Canada: Kluwer Academic Publishers, PO Box 358, Accord Station, Hingham, MA 02018-0358, USA
for all other countries: Kluwer Academic Publishers Group, Distribution Center, PO Box 322, 3300 AH Dordrecht, The Netherlands

British Library Cataloguing in Publication Data

Godfrey, Martin *1956-*
    The hyperlipidaemia handbook.
    1. Man. Blood. Hyperlipidaemia
    I. Title
    616.3997

    ISBN 0-7923-8960-3

Library of Congress Cataloging in Publication Data

Godfrey, Martin, MB ChB
    The hyperlipidaemia handbook / Martin Godfrey ; with a foreword by J. Shepherd.
        p.   cm.
    Includes bibliographical references.
    Includes index.
    ISBN 0-7923-8960-3 (casebound)
    1. Hyperlipidemia-Handbooks, manuals, etc. I. Title.
    [DNLM: 1. Family Practice. 2. Hyperlipidemia.   WD 200.5.H8 G583h]
    RC632.H87G63   1990
    616.3'997-dc20
    DNLM/DLC
    for Library of Congress   90-5234
                                                                        CIP

Copyright

Published in the United Kingdom by Kluwer Academic Publishers, PO Box 55, Lancaster, UK.

Kluwer Academic Publishers BV incorporates the publishing programmes of D. Reidel, Martinus Nijhoff, Dr W. Junk and MTP Press.

Printed in Great Britain by Butler and Tanner Limited, Frome and London.

Contents

Foreword

J. Shepherd

Coronary artery disease, the most important cause of death in the United Kingdom, kills about 200 000 Britons each year. Many victims are struck down out of the blue and in the prime of an active working life. Others survive the first attack but are so debilitated by it that they are compelled to fall back on the efforts of their family and the Social and Health Services for their future survival. The epidemic proportions of the problem and the burden which it places on the community at large has led many health care professionals to reassess their attitudes to heart disease prevention. In the past, the clinician's attention has been directed primarily at the treatment of established ischaemic heart disease rather than focussing on forestalling its appearance by attempting to tackle those life-style habits within the population which appear to predispose to it. A number of recent developments make this approach hard to sustain. First, there is now convincing evidence that action taken against cigarette smoking, hypertension and hypercholesterolaemia offers significant protection to the individual. Secondly, effective and apparently safe antihypertensive and lipid-lowering agents have recently become available to the practicing clinician. Thirdly, developments in computer technology and laboratory equipment manufacture have brought the measurement of coronary risk factors right into the primary health care setting. And, last, but not least, political attitudes towards prevention now favour the enthusiastic general practitioner with an interest in anticipating and averting the development of degenerative diseases like atherosclerosis.

But doctors need more than enthusiasm. What practical steps can be taken to identify the patient at risk and to provide appropriate preventive measures? This handbook offers pragmatic and sound advice straight from the general practitioner's office on how to approach this problem. Designed to focus primarily on hyperlipidaemia, it describes the inherited and environmental factors associated with the condition, and provides practical guidelines for their detection and treatment. It, quite rightly, emphasizes the necessity to employ dietary intervention as the primary approach to lipid lowering, adding drug therapy to this regimen only when the desired effect is not achieved. And the importance of taking concerted action against the other major coronary risk factors is stressed. The publication of this volume provides timely guidance for the prevention of our most prevalent preventable disease.

1
Hyperlipidaemia – is it really a GP's problem?

This chapter contains information on the following:

- the evidence linking high blood cholesterol with coronary heart disease
- the concept of 'normal' and 'ideal' levels of serum cholesterol
- prevalence of hyperlipidaemia in the UK and worldwide
- likelihood of coming across hyperlipidaemia in the GP's surgery

---

Cholesterol is bad for you. This rather bald statement is probably one that most members of the general public would agree with. They don't know that much about it. They've an idea that it's in butter and eggs. But like smoking, alcohol and sex, they've been taught from all manner of sources that it can do you harm.

OK, that's not a bad start. At least the world's health educationists have got it onto the agenda (more so unfortunately in the USA than in Britain). At least people are learning not to take their food for granted. But there is still a yawning gap between what they think they know and what they actually do with that knowledge. The fact that over 150,000 people die every year from heart disease is testament to that.

CHD statistics in UK

* 500 people die every day as a result of CHD
* CHD accounts for over a third of all deaths in men aged between 40 and 70
* 30 per cent of all male deaths are from CHD
* 5000 men below the age of 55 die from CHD each year

So what can be done? How can the population of this country be educated into not killing themselves? The answer to that is long and tortuous, but surely part of it must lie with the medical profession and more specifically with the general practitioner since it is he or she who comes most into contact with people and their health.

1

So, let's look at the opening statement again – cholesterol is bad for you. How many GPs would agree with that? Probably a lot. What else do you know about cholesterol? You know it is a risk factor for the development of coronary heart disease. You know it is present in butter and eggs. But what else do you know?

Obviously there are many GPs who know an awful lot about lipids and their functions in the body, but there are also a probably larger number who know only a little. The study of hyperlipidaemias at medical school was always rather confusing (that Frederickson classification with all its Type I's, Type IIa's and so on was guaranteed to switch off all but the most diligent of scholars), and to be honest it has only been recently that a strong link between cholesterol and CHD has been properly established. Hyperlipidaemia in the 1940s, 50s, 60s and even the 70s was a group of difficult conditions some of which gave interesting physical signs.

Armed with this little piece of honesty, it is hardly surprising that our population doesn't know its polyunsaturates from its elbow. The first job in educating the public must be to educate its teachers – the general practitioners.

QUESTION: CHOLESTEROL IS BAD FOR YOU – TRUE OR FALSE?

Of course it's false. Cholesterol along with all the other substances loosely known as lipids are absolutely essential for life. Cholesterol is an important constituent of all cell membranes and the precursor for all adrenocortical and sex hormones as well as the bile acids. Without it we could not hope to exist.

The question is misleading. It is too much cholesterol that is bad for us, not its existence in the body.

HOW MUCH IS TOO MUCH?

This is the nub of the matter. The determination of what should be the optimal or ideal level of cholesterol in the human body is something that has exercised the minds of clinicians the world over for many years.

In any group of objects the decision as to what is 'normal' and what is 'ideal' must always be a very difficult one. A 5lb bag of potatoes, for example, will contain potatoes of varying shapes and sizes; almost certainly all will be of different weights and none will have the same circumference. So how do we determine what is the normal and what is the ideal weight of a potato in that bag?

Well we could start by weighing each and then dividing the total by the number of potatoes in the sack. That would give use an average weight. Obviously this is not the normal weight since one or two very large or very small potatoes could skew the average in one direction or another, so in order to make allowances for this we must set a range – a normal range with upper and lower limits. A normal potato will therefore be any potato whose weight falls within these limits.

But would we be correct in describing these normal potatoes as having an ideal weight? Obviously not. For a start this is only one 5lb bag. The average in other bags may be totally different thus what is normal in one bag may be very abnormal in another. Secondly the term ideal is a very loose one; ideal for what we must ask. The terms 'normal' and 'ideal' are not necessarily synonymous (in fact they are only rarely the same).

The decision as to what is ideal is thus complex – subjective judgements and experimentation must come into play. The ideal potato for making chips, for instance, might be much bigger than is normal. The ideal for making roast potatoes might be smaller than normal.

All this might sound a bit obvious and perhaps irrelevant to general practice, but let's just look at how in the past these terms have been terribly mixed up when it came to decisions about what was normal and what was ideal in blood cholesterol levels.

Not so long ago it was the practice of most laboratories in the UK to quote reference ranges for blood cholesterol that had been set arbitrarily at the mean serum value of samples taken plus or minus two standard deviations. This resulted in labs sending clinicians results with reference ranges that now seem ludicrously wide. Upper levels as high as 7.2 mmol per litre were not unknown. Only the top 5 or 10 per cent of samples were therefore taken to be abnormal.

Unfortunately as we now know these were anything but normal and certainly not ideal levels. Let's take the analogy of bags of potatoes and compare the average readings in the UK with those of another 'bag' of people, the Japanese.

In Japan a 'normal' range might well produce an upper limit of perhaps as little as 5 mmol per litre – the average Japanese and the average Briton thus had vastly different amounts of cholesterol coursing through their veins. A Japanese with a cholesterol level of only 5.3 mmol per litre could thus be branded as 'abnormal' in Japan, but even with a level of 6.3 mmol per litre he would still be considered normal in the UK (in fact 6.3 mmol is the normal level for most adult men in this country). Considering that there can be little or no physiological differences in lipid metabolism between these two races something must be terribly wrong (Figure 1).

The problem of course was that there was no ideal level of cholesterol, only national average ranges. It took many years and many large trials to establish what that ideal should be.

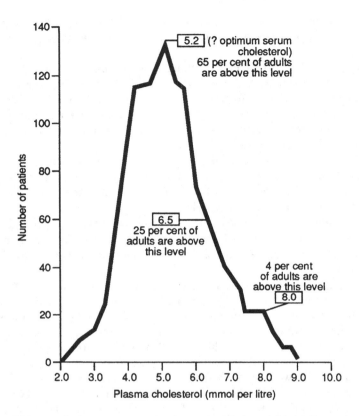

Figure 1. This graph, based on results from the National Lipid Screening Project, show that levels of cholesterol are distributed continuously in the population, thus 'normal' levels are essentially arbitrary

WHAT IS THE IDEAL SERUM CHOLESTEROL LEVEL?

Since population averages vary so much it has been extremely difficult to set any one international level above which a person might be considered to be in danger of CHD. For many years the British Cardiac Society advised that anyone with a level above 6.5 mmol per litre should be considered for therapy. Other countries set different national levels.

Only after a number of large studies, most notably the American Multiple Risk Factor Intervention Trial (MRFIT), and various consensus panels had reported their results did an ideal level become accepted. **This level is 5.2 mmol per litre** (Figure 2).

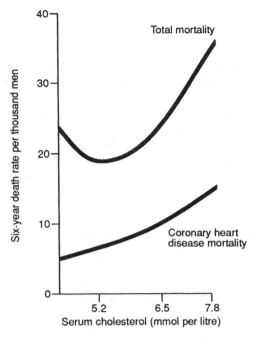

Figure 2. Cholesterol and CHD Mortality (MRFIT Study). Trials have shown that total mortality is lowest when serum cholesterol is 5.2 mmol per litre

The MRFIT trial in particular showed that at this level of cholesterol the total mortality of a group of 350,000 men, measured in terms of the six-year death rate per 1000 men, was at its lowest. Above (and below) this level the total mortality began to rise again.

WHAT DOES THIS MEAN FOR THE AVERAGE GP?

Put simply it means that over 50 per cent of the patients on your list will have higher than ideal levels of cholesterol in their blood. And about 1 per cent – roughly 20 individuals is an average list size – will have very severely elevated cholesterol levels.

These statistics were underlined recently by a large survey carried out in the UK by the National Lipid Screening Project. The research team examined the plasma cholesterol levels in both men and women aged between 20 and 59 in Glasgow, Leicester, London and Oxford.

Their results showed that not only were the distributions of cholesterol levels similar in both men and women, but that an astonishing 65 per cent of adults were above the supposed optimum of 5.2 mmol per litre.

GPs have a massive problem on their hands

Before moving on, it is worth noting that total mortality rose again in the MRFIT study as total serum cholesterol levels dropped below 4.0 mmol per litre. This increased mortality is due to neoplasms, mainly colorectal cancer.

Although many studies have shown that this increase in the incidence of cancer is not due to lipids, many experts have persisted in advising that levels of cholesterol should not be pushed too low. Recent research, however, has shown that it is the cancers that produce the low cholesterol, not the other way round: rapidly growing tumours need as much cholesterol as they can get to form new cell walls, so it is not surprising that levels are low in these patients.

There is no risk in having low cholesterol levels.

THE LINK BETWEEN SERUM CHOLESTEROL AND CORONARY HEART DISEASE

So far we have established that there is a relationship between high levels of serum cholesterol and mortality. What we have not yet proven is that cholesterol plays a part in CHD mortality.

This may sound a bit pedantic, but in truly scientific terms, it has to be. It is no use getting 65 per cent of your practice to change their eating habits if after a few years someone pops up and says "Sorry, we got it wrong – cholesterol is OK after all". The patients would never trust you again.

Surprisingly, any number of things can be correlated with the risk of getting CHD. Personality, positions in higher management, even car ownership has been shown to have a link in one study or another. The key is to find factors whose effects cannot be explained in terms of their effects on the others.

This has been established in the cases of high blood pressure, smoking, obesity, age and gender (see Chapter 2). The question is, can the link be established for cholesterol?

POPULATION STUDIES

Some of the strongest and most powerful evidence comes from epidemiological studies of CHD mortality rates in different countries.

Nations which eat a typical Northern European, high-fat diet all have the very highest levels of CHD. Scotland and Northern Ireland head the list together with Finland (Figure 3).

Nations on the other hand which eat very little saturated fat, such as Japan, or a lot of monounsaturated fats (olive oil), such as those countries surrounding the Mediterranean, have much lower levels of CHD.

Table 1. International comparisons of CHD

	Rate per 100,000	
	Men	Women
N. Ireland	341	93
Scotland	336	103
Finland	317	51
USSR	294	85
USA	197	61
Denmark	199	50
Sweden	183	35
W. Germany	164	35
Israel	159	49
E. Germany	145	35
Belgium	131	31
Italy	115	23
Spain	89	17
France	79	13
Japan	29	9

Source: *WHO Statistical Tables*, 1989

Further confirmatory evidence that diet rather than something intrinsic to the national metabolism is involved comes from studies of Japanese nationals who settled on the west coast of America after the war.

These people rapidly dropped their old national diets of fish and rice and switched to a much more fat-rich one of hamburgers and french fries. Before long their serum cholesterol levels began to mirror those of all other Californians and inevitably their levels off CHD also began to rise becoming close to those of the rest of America.

Another population of Japanese who moved only as far as Hawaii – and only half-heartedly adopted the American lifestyle – developed only slightly higher levels of CHD than did their native Japanese counterparts. Western diet, not Western nationality, is thus the link.

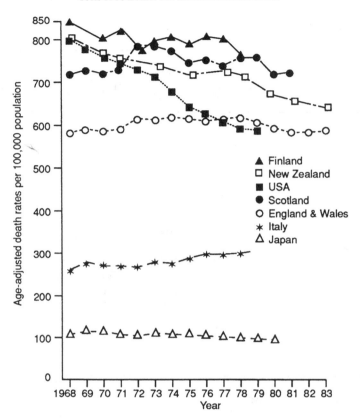

Figure 3. Trends in CHD mortality. Coronary heart disease mortality 1968–82 in selected countries (men aged 35–74 years). (Data from Marmot, 1985, Acta Med. Scand. suppl., 701, 58–65)

LARGE INTERVENTION STUDIES

But population studies are not enough. There are so many variables that it is very difficult to confidently point at cholesterol as being the CHD culprit – it could just as easily have been a variety of other things either singly or in combination.

What clinched the medical world's general acceptance that cholesterol was a major risk factor in CHD were the recent results of two large intervention studies, one in America, the other in Finland (see Appendix II).

The first was the Lipid Research Clinics (LRC) Trial. This was conducted in several centres around the USA and recruited almost 4000 middle-aged men to take part. None of these men had any evidence of CHD and yet each, despite attempts to modify their diet, had a very high level of cholesterol. Their average

8

cholesterol was 7.2 mmol per litre, a level that put them into the top 2.5 per cent in the country.

All were randomised to take either the lipid-lowering drug cholestyramine or placebo.

After seven years (in 1983) the trial was concluded. A number of the men taking cholestyramine had failed to keep up with the treatment (having to take six sachets a day led to poor compliance; the drug also produces a lot of GI symptoms); nevertheless these were still asigned to the total treatment group when the results were finally analysed. (This accounts for the fact that there was only an 8 per cent difference in cholesterol levels between those on the drug and those on placebo.)

The effect of even this lowering of cholesterol on coronary morbidity was marked – there was a 15 to 40 per cent reduction in all cardiovascular end points. And in those men who continued to take the six sachets for the full seven years a 25 per cent cholesterol lowering was achieved leading to a massive 50 per cent drop in coronary morbidity and mortality.

These results were greeted with a good deal of euphoria when they were announced (they even made the front page of *Time* magazine). But there were still sceptics. In particular a number of experts argued that although these figures showed irrefutably that lowering cholesterol in people with severely raised levels could indeed reduce their chances of having a heart attack, they could not be extrapolated out to prove that lowering cholesterol in everyone's diet would lessen the chances of heart disease. The medical establishment continued to watch and wait.

The sceptics were finally won over in 1986 when the results of the Helsinki Heart Study were published. This trial which was started in Finland in 1981 again involved 4000 middle aged men whose average total cholesterol level was 7.4 mmol per litre. They were randomly assigned to take either the lipid-lowering drug gemfibrazil twice daily or placebo.

After five years there was a 34 per cent reduction in cardiac events in the drug-treated group compared with those who were taking placebo and a 37 per cent reduction in non-fatal myocardial infarction. The cholesterol level was lowered 10 per cent by the drug.

These studies show that it is cholesterol that is having an effect on CHD and that, like smoking and high blood pressure, serum cholesterol is an independent risk factor for the disease. Overall these two studies show that a 1 per cent fall in serum cholesterol levels will result in a two per cent fall in CHD.

To be honest there are still those who criticise the cholesterol hypothesis. There are some who are still dubious about the overall benefits of lowering cholesterol pointing out that in no major study has the overall mortality (as opposed to the mortality due to CHD) been shown to decrease.

In both the Helsinki and LRC trials, roughly the same number of men died from all causes, including cancer, in both placebo and drug-treated groups. Lowering the level of cholesterol thus lessens the chances of CHD, but it doesn't, on present evidence, do much for your overall chances of dying from something else.

It is worth remembering, however, that these studies were designed specifically to look at cardiac morbidity and mortality not overall mortality. More trials must be carried out to fully elucidate this conundrum. It seems likely that once trials such as these are followed up for long enough (say 20 years), overall mortality will also be shown to be reduced.

2
Cholesterol in perspective as a coronary heart disease risk factor

---

This chapter contains information on the following:

- CHD risk factors – smoking, hypertension, obesity, diabetes, age and sex
- Other lipid risk factors – LDL, HDL and triglyceride
- Importance of risk factor interaction

Since it is still not possible to point at an individual and say "this person is going to have a heart attack", medical science has had to make do with detecting a series of factors, the presence of which will imply a greater than average risk of a heart attack occurring.

As we have seen in Chapter 1, a high level of serum cholesterol is one of these factors. But as we all know it is not the only one. Smoking, high blood pressure, obesity, age, sex and diabetes all play their part. Lets have a look at each and then see what bearing they have on the serum cholesterol.

SMOKING

Cigarette smoking is generally acknowledged to be the single most preventable cause of premature death in the Western World. Among other things it can lead to the development of emphysema, lung cancer and of course heart disease (Figure 4) and contributes to the exacerbation of asthma, peptic ulcer disease, gastric reflux, and much more. Faced with this list it's a wonder any government permits it to be practised.

Be that as it may, smoking is a fact and as such must be faced squarely by every family physician. Happily smoking is on the decline, but it is still practiced widely by men and women of all ages. Oddly it is the women who have found it hardest to quit. Smoking rates are decreasing more slowly in women than in men, and, in the younger age groups, smoking in women is actually on the increase.

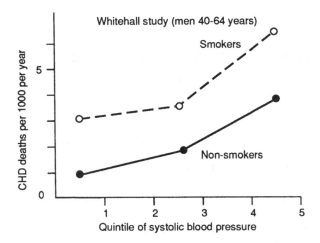

Figure 4. Smoking and systolic blood-pressure as risk factors for CHD. From the Whitehall study of British civil servants (Data from Reid et al. *(1976).* Lancet, ii, *979–984)*

Talking specifically about heart disease now, it has been shown that there is a direct, linear relationship between the number of cigarettes smoked per day, the number of years that this has been happening and the development of CHD: regular smoking nearly doubles the risk of cardiovascular mortality and almost triples the risk of sudden death.

There are almost certainly many mechanisms by which smoking helps produce CHD. Abnormally high levels of carboxyhaemoglobin lowers the overall oxygen carrying ability of the blood thus leaving the endothelium more susceptible to injury, the blood is also more likely to clot, lipid levels are altered and there is a greater likelihood of arrhythmias developing. This cocktail increases the chances of CHD even into the 60s and 70s (although the relative risk does decrease somewhat the older you get).

Unlike its effects on other diseases such as lung cancers and respiratory problems, stopping smoking quickly lessens a patient's chances of having CHD.

Current evidence suggests that after as little as 12 months the relative risk of developing CHD can be as low as that in non-smokers in some individuals. Even if some degree of coronary artery disease exists already, stopping smoking can still be beneficial. In one study (the Coronary Artery Surgery Study) the rate of fatal myocardial infarction was 7.9 per cent in patients with CHD who continued to smoke, yet only 4.4 per cent in similar patients who stopped.

In view of statistics like these it is obviously very worthwhile for doctors to try to get their patients to stop. It has been shown in a number of studies that a doctor's advice on its own is an extremely powerful and effective method of getting patients to give up. A number of organisations, most notably the Health Education Authority and the anti-smoking group 'ASH' have some very sophisticated tools available that can be used by GPs to stop patients smoking – patient leaflets, posters and so on. These can be used in a co-ordinated campaign using the practice nurse and all the partners to reduce smoking in the practice.

Oddly, despite its well-known adverse effects, very few GPs keep a note of whether a patient is a smoker or non-smoker. Investment in a set of stickers or even just a marker pen to label the notes of smokers would be a useful first step.

HYPERTENSION

As with cigarette smoking, a raised blood pressure shows a near linear relationship to the risk of developing CHD. This is true at all ages and for both sexes. Despite the fact that treatment is based on the diastolic pressure, the absolute risk of CHD is related slightly more strongly to systolic blood pressure.

By and large the all-cause mortality rate rises by 1 per cent for each millimeter rise in blood pressure. CHD is by far the most common clinical manifestation of high blood pressure.

When it comes to treatment there has been much controversy as to its efficacy. As a result of many large and very thorough trials, it is clear that reducing blood pressure has a positive effect in relieving stroke, renal failure and congestive heart disease in men with a diastolic blood pressure above 105 mmHg. However the evidence is not so strong for myocardial infarction – particularly in mild to moderate hypertension where the risk of drug therapy could be argued to outweigh the risk of hypertension itself.

Until proved otherwise, reducing the blood pressure will help to prevent stroke but will not have a great effect on the likelihood of a patient having a heart attack.

Drugs, such as diuretics, β-blockers, calcium antagonists and ACE inhibitors are obviously effective in reducing blood pressure and there is no room here to go into their use in any further detail. In mild hypertension, however, a number of non-pharmacological methods have been shown to be very effective in reducing blood pressure. These include weight reduction (by far the most effective), biofeedback, relaxation techniques and so on.

OBESITY

Although obesity has for many years been associated with other CHD risk factors such as hypertension and diabetes, it is only recently that it has been shown to be an independent risk factor.

The key to assessing whether someone is obese or not is to establish whether or not they are 'overweight', the criteria for which is the body mass index (weight/height^2) and the standard age-to-weight charts used by insurance companies.

The exact link between obesity and CHD is not absolutely clear, although it is thought to be linked to the development of a relative insulin resistance and therefore an abnormal glucose tolerance. One particular group, the so-called syndrome-X sufferers, tend to have a very high incidence of CHD and typically sport a 'spare tyre', mildly altered glucose tolerance and slightly raised lipids. Younger patients with spare tyres should be monitored closely for signs of CHD although any young patient who is obese should be strongly counselled to lose weight, since life-long obesity leads to a 50 per cent increase in the death rate from CHD.

A reduction in weight, even to levels way above what may be thought of as normal for the build, can dramatically reduce a clutch of risk factors.

Weight reduction is naturally based upon a calorie-controlled diet. The appropriate degree of calorie restriction can be aproximated by subtracting 500 to 1000 kcal from the patient's estimated daily maintenance requirements (12 kcal per lb).

Exercise and some form of behaviour modification are also essential if any weight reduction is to become permanent.

DIABETES

Individuals with an impaired glucose tolerance or frank diabetes mellitus are very much at risk from CHD. Diabetes roughly doubles the chances of CHD mortality and CHD is the most common complication of the disease. For some reason it is a more potent risk in women than it is in men.

As mentioned above, insulin resistance seems to be the key, although the exact mechanism by which atherosclerosis is linked to this is still not altogether clear. Certainly lipid metabolism is also altered and this is reflected in a diabetic's lipid profile (triglycerides for example tend to be very high).

Studies have not confirmed that the risk of CHD is reduced to any significant extent by normalising a patient's glucose tolerance.

OTHER RISK FACTORS

Age is the most obvious. CHD increases with age in both sexes, but in women it tends to be lower before the menopause, after which womens' rates catch up (suggesting that female sex hormones have a protective effect against CHD).

Other factors seem to have a strong link, but have not yet been proven to be independent risk factors: behaviour patterns, particularly that known as 'Type A', characterised by extreme competitiveness, impatience, aggressiveness, rapid movements and so on, has been linked with CHD – anger and hostility seem to be the most important components; gout and hyperuricaemia have long been thought to be associated; alcohol when taken in moderation seems to protect against heart disease, but higher levels seem to increase the likelihood of the disease; a high level of fibrinogen is also considered to be a strong candidate for independent risk factor status.

Undoubtedly, CHD does seem to run in some families – particularly that causing myocardial infarction at an early age. Presumably there is an interaction here between environmental factors and some genetic predisposition.

HYPERLIPIDAEMIA

High levels of circulating cholesterol certainly play an important part in the development of atherosclerotic plaques; they are therefore directly linked to the incidence of myocardial infarction. A description of the process of plaque formation is to be found in Appendix I.

The measurement of the total amount of cholesterol in the blood is not however as precise an indicator of CHD risk as we might like. This is because serum cholesterol is not a homogenous material in the blood stream. Cholesterol is insoluble; thus in order to travel around the body it must be combined with other lipids (phospholipids and triglyceride) and proteins (apolipoproteins) to form a series of what are called lipoproteins.

Lipoproteins can be classified on the basis of their density after ultracentrifugation into a number of types, namely chylomicrons – very low density lipoproteins (VLDL); low density lipoproteins (LDL) and high density lipoproteins (HDL) – a full description of which is not warranted here but which can be found in Appendix I.

LDL cholesterol delivers the bulk (about 70 per cent) of the body's circulating cholesterol to the tissues themselves and is known to play a key role in atheroma formation. Not surprisingly LDL measurement is held to be the key to accurate CHD risk prediction and supersedes the more crude total cholesterol levels as an independent risk factor.

Unfortunately LDL cannot be measured directly in most laboratories and must be derived from the rather difficult calculation:

$$LDL = \text{total cholesterol} - (HDL + \text{triglyceride}/2.19)$$

(This is known as the Friedewald formula and is only accurate provided triglyceride concentrations do not exceed 4.5 mmol per litre.)

Because of the difficulty in calculating LDL, few clinical studies have been carried out specifically to meaure the correlation between CHD and LDL; there is thus no internationally accepted normal range. Levels above 3.5 mmol per litre appear to attract greater risk if other risk factors are present.

HDL is also an important risk factor in its own right according to most studies (including the Helsinki heart study). Its job is to ferry cholesterol from the circulation into the liver for elimination in the bile; thus high levels confer a beneficial effect and low levels, particularly if below 0.9 mmol per litre, confer a higher risk of CHD.

Lastly triglyceride: high levels of triglyceride will certainly increase the likelihood of a patient developing pancreatitis, but opinions differ as to the importance of this lipid as an independent risk factor in CHD. It may be that high levels of triglyceride are important, but as yet they have not been shown to cause atherosclerosis. Triglycerides must exert their effects in some other way.

One answer may have come from a recent Swedish study which has shown evidence that triglyceride levels are related to myocardial infarction but not to the development of angina. It may be that this lipid exerts its effect through another agent such as fibrinogen, enhancing the blood's ability to form clots.

In general, if the level of triglyceride is above 2.3 mmol per litre and the HDL level is low, then there is a strong link with CHD.

THE INTERACTION BETWEEN RISK FACTORS

CHD risk factors rarely exist in isolation and they always have an effect on each other. The combination of smoking and high cholesterol levels is a particularly lethal combination for instance; add in hypertension and the risk is multiplied many fold.

At the end of the day, cholesterol, LDL, HDL and triglycerides are all just laboratory investigations no matter how high they may be. Any plan of action must be based on a broad knowledge of all the risk factors present in one patient.

3
Finding your patient

This chapter contains information on the following:

- The arguments for and against testing the whole population's cholesterol levels
- The arguments for and against selective testing in high-risk groups
- Details of the King's Fund Consensus Statement on 'Blood Cholesterol Measurement in the Prevention of Coronary Heart Disease'
- Details of the Standing Medical Advisory Committee report

So far we have established that there does seem to be a link between high levels of serum cholesterol and heart disease and that an awful lot of people in this country – about 60 per cent – have levels above what is thought to be safe (5.2 mmol per litre). What, as a society, should we be doing about it and more specifically how does the GP play a part?

To be honest this is not an easy question to answer. Ever since the link between cholesterol and CHD was finally established, physicians, dieticians, epidemiologists and politicians the world over have been fighting over what exactly should be done.

As yet no-one has come up with an acceptable or definitive strategy, but these are early days. Every country has developed, or is in the process of developing its own methods for dealing with the problem, their decision based both on the prevelence of CHD in that country and the cost of setting up some sort of nationwide programme to deal with it. A number of countries have adopted completely different approaches and only time and a few wheelbarrows full of statistics will tell who is right and who wrong.

Basically there are two arguments: screen the entire population so that everyone is aware of their cholesterol level, or screen only those at highest risk while simultaneously introducing some form of national policy to promote a healthier diet.

MASS SCREENING: THE ARGUMENT FOR

Mass screening is on the face of it quite a logical argument particularly in countries such as Britain where a large proportion of the population has high levels.

The Americans and a number of European countries have opted for this approach, (the American National Heart Lung and Blood Institute in particular being strongly in favour of it) and already six out of ten Americans know their 'number'. Officials hope that in time this proportion will increase.

Those that support mass screening argue that by telling patients what their cholesterol level is you are giving them the chance to take responsibility for their own health. Patients with high levels will have a powerful incentive to change their eating habits and even those with normal levels may be encouraged to eat more sensibly.

What is more, since patients with high levels of cholesterol often have no outward signs that this is so, mass screening is the only way that medicine will detect the many thousands of individuals who have some form of hyper-lipidaemia. Without blanket screening these patients are at real risk of falling prey to an avoidable heart attack.

How would mass screening be achieved?

In the USA, mass screening has become an overnight sensation. Private companies have set up screening operations at a variety of locations including supermarkets and drug stores, and this complements the work of hospitals and family physicians who are attempting to screen as many patients as possible.

Naturally patients in the USA pay a fee. This is fine in the local hospitals, but unfortunately in many of the small supermarket and drug store operations there is often little or no advice or counselling to go with the test, making its benefit in these situations somewhat dubious.

In Britain no decision has yet been made to go for mass screening (although a parliamentary subcommittee – the Standing Medical Advisory Committee – has been looking into the question – see below). So while some prevaricate and others back selective screening (see below), a number of organisations have taken it upon themselves to start the ball rolling unilaterally.

It is the pharmacists in particular who have really taken the idea of mass screening to their bosom. Emboldened by the 1986 White Paper: 'Promoting Better Health' which argued an extended role in health promotion and prevention for Britain's 11,000 community pharmacists, and helped by the development of a number of quite sophisticated and relatively cheap desktop diagnostic machines, the pharmacists' representative body, the Pharmaceutical Services Negotiating Committee, in 1989 launched a pilot study of High Street cholesterol testing.

This 12-week study took place in pharmacies in Coventry, Sheffield, Newcastle upon Tyne and Nottingham. Patients were charged £6.00 and in return they were given a finger-prick blood test and a form which recorded the result, together with a guide to the interpretation of cholesterol measurements in terms of the action required of them. Results were provided in triplicate – one for the pharmacy, one for the patient and one for the patient's GP should the level be above 6.5 mmol per litre. One-to-one counselling and advice was also available, the 'consultation' taking in all about 30 minutes.

One very important thing to note about the pharmacist's experience with lipid testing is that it is extremely popular with the public, so popular in fact that it has prompted the PSNC to consider extending the service nationwide. There is no doubt that if it were generally available, screening would be just as much a hit in the UK as it was in the USA.

Meanwhile, as the pharmacists and the medical profession consider what to do next, the prominent health shop chain Holland and Barrett saw 17,000 patients in just four weeks when it started a similar scheme in its 90 stores up and down the country. A private company called Health First set the thing up for them and charges £5 for the test (although for this you don't get much in the way of privacy or counselling).

More and more pharmacies are now beginning to fork out the £3000 needed to buy these new cholesterol testing machines, so whether the medical profession as a whole likes it or not, some form of mass screening seems inevitable in the coming years.

The Americans are for it, the public seems to want it, and even august bodies such as the European Atherosclerosis Society, the British Hyperlipidaemia Association and the Family Heart Association say it should be introduced. Why then are we not screening the whole population, especially since we have the highest levels of heart disease in the world?

MASS SCREENING: THE ARGUMENT AGAINST

There are many reasons, none of them clear cut, but at the end of the day, it is currently the 'de facto' policy in Britain to eschew mass screening for a more selective approach. The reasons for this are as follows:

First, those that oppose mass screening point out that one of the principal reasons it is performed – to create in patients an incentive to lower their own cholesterol through sensible eating – is patently unproven. There is little or no evidence to confirm that patients given their cholesterol levels will do anything very much about it in the long term. In fact giving them their 'number' may be counterproductive – especially in those that have low or borderline readings. A normal level is usually interpreted by the patient as a green light for indulging in all the foods he or she may up until then have avoided. Giving a patient his number may make them eat more fat, not less.

Rather than complement other strategies to improve the population's health, mass screening could actually destroy them. A national 'healthy eating' campaign, a measure recommended by many bodies, could be particularly hard hit.

Proponents of mass screening of course point out that those who take the blood must be trained in counselling patients as to what foods they should eat and what they should do to keep their level of cholesterol down. But unfortunately, as has been the case in the USA, all too often screening is set up as a money making exercise with little or no back up. As such it can do more harm than good.

Another of the critics' main arguments centres on the fact that simply testing someone's cholesterol and nothing else is next to useless. The other major independent CHD risk factors must be assessed as well.

The reason for this was mentioned in the last chapter, but cannot be said too often: CHD is a multifactorial condition; analysed alone, cholesterol is simply a laboratory result (albeit an important one) and that is all. It is just one side of a many-sided picture – smoking, high blood pressure, obesity, age, sex and diabetes all play a part and must be looked for.

Take for example, the studies carried out in the 350,000 or so men screened in the MRFIT trial in the USA. Results from this trial show that the CHD risk attributable to a high level of serum cholesterol in men aged 35–45, who do not smoke and have a low blood pressure, is minimal.

On the other hand a man in the same age group who smoked, had high blood pressure and also had a high serum cholesterol would be at very grave risk. The risk is thus relative and must be properly assessed before any decision can be made about management. This sort of assessment is patently impossible to do as a routine screening exercise for the whole population.

Finally we come to cost. There are no accurate figures obviously, but some assumptions can be made about the cost of mass screening. For a start, an approach which gives every person a cholesterol figure plus information about what is normal and what is not and nothing else, will rapidly trigger a massive demand for treatment.

Since drug therapy can cost in excess of £500 per year and may have to go on for a life-time, it is not hard to see that if large numbers start getting treated in this way, the total bill will be astronomical. Some estimates see the NHS drugs bill rising by 20 per cent as a result – that is over £400 million. And then there is the cost of the testing itself and of paying for the counselling that would be needed. No one dares guess at how much the final total might be. Unfortunately accurate cost benefit analyses are still awaited.

SELECTIVE SCREENING OF HIGH-RISK PATIENTS: THE ARGUMENT FOR

So what is proposed in its place? The British Medical Association, the British Heart Foundation and the Coronary Prevention Group, together with the vast bulk of interested medical opinion in this country, believe that the answer in the UK, given its huge population burden and limited NHS funds, is selective screening of high-risk patients followed by the opportunistic testing of the rest of the population, combined with a national campaign to promote healthier eating.

These sentiments were strongly backed in June 1989 by a consensus conference of Britain's top lipid experts organised by the independent charity, the King's Fund.

The King's Fund panel took evidence from many sources, finally releasing the following recommendations at the end of three days of contemplation:

1. The most important and effective way to reduce CHD is through a national food and health strategy to reduce the general level of blood cholesterol in the population.

2. Clear and consistent information about risk factors and the means of reducing those which are affected, by changes in individual behaviour, especially smoking and diet, should be disseminated.

3. Everyone should be encouraged and advised to make appropriate dietary changes.

4. Mass measurement of blood cholesterol levels in the population is not justified.

5. CHD risk assessment should be made on the basis of factors other than measured blood cholesterol levels. If one or more major risk factor is present then we recommend testing.

6. Cholesterol measurement should never occur without direct access to advice and counselling services.

7. Only when dietary changes are seen to be ineffective or inappropriate should drug therapy be considered.

8. The initiation of drug treatment requires specialist medical advice.

9. All cholesterol lowering drugs should be subject to adequate evaluation and monitoring.

The King's Fund recommendations are not set in stone. A number of its recommendations, such as the suggestion that all drug treatment should be started by specialists, are highly contentious. And their main recommendation for a national food and health policy is still a long way off. But generally they endorse what is now the 'establishment' view that lipids should only be measured in those at high risk of CHD. This is enough.

SELECTIVE SCREENING OF HIGH-RISK PATIENTS: THE ARGUMENT AGAINST

It is worth just finally looking at the few criticisms that can still be levelled at selective screening.

The most obvious is that selective screening will not easily pick up the 1 in 500 patients who have unrecognised and asymptomatic hyperlipidaemia. At present we are picking up under 10 per cent of them in the UK whereas the mass screening going on in the US and parts of Europe is resulting in the detection of between 40 and 60 per cent. It may be in the future that the routine testing of neonatal cord blood will act as a safety net, but as yet in the UK that is still some way off and what is more it tends to be innaccurate.

It is argued that since all patients will have to be invited to attend their doctor's surgery every three years under the new contract, a good proportion could ultimately be picked up by opportunistic testing. This will obviously depend on the individual GP's time and enthusiasm.

The other major criticism is more of an observation. It is surprising that countries such as the USA should adopt a scheme we in Britain seem to have rejected. Obviously only time will show who is right.

To some extent this difference in approach is a repetition of what happened in the 1970s with hypertension. At that time the USA decided to institute a vigorous national campaign against this condition, while in Britain there were doubts and no such campaign appeared.

It is interesting to note that in America where the public's awareness about hypertension and cholesterol is greater, the level of CHD has crept down significantly over the last few years. In Britain it has only recently begun to dip.

SMAC REPORT

The Standing Medical Advisory Committee (SMAC) on blood cholesterol testing published its recommendations to both the government and the medical profession in July 1990.

Unfortunately their conclusions were not as helpful as many had hoped. However the SMAC did confirm that "some form of opportunistic blood cholesterol testing and treatment programme does have the potential to make a cost-effective contribution to CHD prevention while others are likely to perform less well". They suggest that CHD risk factors should be identified and priority for cholesterol testing given to those at high overall risk.

They also say that they consider that "inviting members of defined target populations to attend for blood cholesterol testing is unlikely to make a cost-effective contribution in situations where a programme of opportunistic testing is already established".

Commercial testing, they say, should be monitored and have codes of practice in order that there would be appropriate quality control of the machines used and counselling afterwards. They say that all testing should be under medical supervision.

The government decided, on receipt of this report, to distribute it to other bodies for consultation. Its recommendations have not been adopted as official policy.

CHD RISK SCORING

Before moving on to the nuts and bolts of what the GP should actually do in his or her practice it is worth just touching on one final alternative strategy for picking up patients at risk of CHD – that is to not bother with the cholesterol measurement at all.

Clinical epidemiologist Professor Gerry Shaper, from the Royal Free Hospital in London, has for some time been advocating that those who are trying to prevent CHD should investigate a patient's CHD risk factors simply by history and examination and use these to calculate what he calls a 'risk score'. Cholesterol testing he says is of limited value.

Professor Shaper's scoring system is calculated as follows:

Smoking: number of years spent smoking × 7.5

+

Blood Pressure: systolic blood pressure (average of two readings) × 4.5

+

Diabetes: if a diabetic add 150

+

Angina: if current angina add 150

+

Family history: if parent died of 'heart trouble' add 80

A score of over 1000 marks the cut-off point above which a patient becomes 'high risk'. According to Professor Shaper's research more than half (54 per cent) of the major CHD events are likely to take place during five years of follow up after this screening.

Measuring the cholesterol level and taking an ECG would, he says, increase the score's predictive value to only 59 per cent – a marginal increase which he thinks makes cholesterol screening unwarranted.

4

Finding your patient in general practice

This chapter contains information on the following:

- High risk groups
- Opportunistic screening
- Starting general practice screening
- The practice CHD prevention clinic
- The practice nurse
- Patient questionnaire
- Children and the elderly

So far we have established that there is a link between high levels of serum cholesterol and CHD and that in the UK the most effective way of finding these patients is to screen selectively the groups of patients who are at highest risk, and to test other patients opportunistically.

First let us define our terms. What is meant by 'high risk'?

High-risk groups

- Patients with a history of CHD, especially when it is presented before the age of 60
- Patients with a family history of hyperlipidaemia
- Patients under 40 with xanthomas or with xanthelasma or corneal arcus (see Figure 9, p. 79)
- Patients with other risk factors such as   – hypertension
         – smoking
         – diabetes
         – obesity

In theory, these patients should be targeted and their cholesterol level measured.

Opportunistic testing

Opportunistic testing, i.e. testing a patient's blood cholesterol as part of consultation not specifically made for this purpose, could in theory be carried out in all patients between the ages of 25 and 65 (the value of testing children and the elderly on any routine basis is highly debatable).

Suitable patients could include:
- All new patients
- Patients coming for a medical
- Patients attending a specially organised health promotion clinic
- Patients attending for their three-yearly check
- Patients who ask for a test

TURNING THEORY INTO PRACTICE

Now we come to the hard part. It is all very well conducting fancy trials, conducting consensus conferences, producing statistics and the like. In the end, however, someone has got to sit down and do these things. That person, judging by the huge numbers of people we have been talking about and the amount of information that is needed, can only be the GP.

For the purposes of this book we will assume that the reader is to every intents and purposes an 'average GP'. That means you have the best of intentions as far as your patients' health is concerned; you have constructed your own age–sex register and have tried to do something to order the notes so that at least everything is in the right order and that the letters and investigations are kept in a separate bundle in the Lloyd George envelope.

You do not however have an accurate disease index or summary card of each patient's major complaints over the years, nor have you organised any special health promotion clinics, but with the arrival of the new contract you are thinking hard about it.

You are planning to get a computer but you haven't got one yet.

Should you be an average GP or close to it you will be well aware of the fact that to screen your patients will be anything but easy:

1. You have no overall record of which patients have the above high-risk conditions, so you can't just summon them all down to the surgery. All information about CHD risk factors, hypertension and so on, is all embedded in the individual notes.

2. Some of the information you are sure you haven't even recorded – smoking for instance. Patients will not usually volunteer the fact that they smoke unless it is pertinent to the consultation (why should they?); thus unless it has been asked about directly there will be no record of it in the notes.

And what about the family history? If the parents live outside your practice, it is very unlikely you will have any record that they are no longer alive let alone have any idea of what they died from.

Unless you are some sort of medical dynamo, your raw material for starting to screen will be very poor. How in that case can you start screening in the practice?

Well for a start it needs planning. It's no use going down to the surgery one afternoon and saying 'I think I'll start screening my patients for high CHD risk today!'. You have to make definite decisions about who will do what, when it will be done and of course how.

WHO WILL DO WHAT?

There aren't too many choices really. Either you do it yourself and each partner individually tries to pick out his own high-risk patients as they come in at random through the door. Alternatively you could employ a practice nurse to help (see below).

WHEN WILL IT BE DONE

Either you can try to squeeze this into your normal surgery hours or you can create time each week to deal with the problem and devote your attention to it properly. Alternatively your practice nurse and practice manager/receptionists could do most of the initial work. In practice the latter is the most sensible solution.

HOW CAN THIS BE ACHIEVED?

I) Those who want an easy way out might, as mentioned above, consider finding their high-risk patients simply by dealing with them as they come through the door for their usual appointment. This might sound easy, but it has a number of drawbacks:

a) To do it properly would mean scanning through the whole of every 25- to 60-year-old's notes as they come through the door: checking if they are hypertensive, have a family history of premature infarction and so on.

b) Much of the information you need has never been written into the notes.

c) You may never see many of the patients who are at highest risk. Young and middle-aged men, for instance, are the least likely to just pop down to the surgery. Naturally they will have to be seen eventually as part of their 3-year check, but this could mean that the job takes an awful long time.

Faced with these problems the GP who opts for this highly opportunistic approach has two alternatives – either give up since he or she will miss so many patients that the exercise is hardly worth doing, or find some way of filling in the blanks in your knowledge when the patient arrives.

The best way to do this is to get your patients to fill out a short questionnaire. The aim of the exercise is to fill in the gaps in your knowledge. The following is a pro-forma:

Name
Age
Sex
Weight
Height
Smoker or non-smoker (if yes how many)
Alcohol intake per week (give range)
Details of any medication
Diabetes?
Do you know if you have high blood pressure and when was it last tested
Have you ever had a heart attack or angina
Any family history of early heart attack (below the age of 50)

This questionnaire can either be used by the GP or the practice nurse when the patient is being interviewed or, better still, it can be filled in by the patients themselves before seeing the doctor. In some practices, question-naires of this sort are left out in the waiting room and patients encouraged via posters on the walls to fill them in.

Such an approach has proved so popular in some health centres that separate appointments have to be made for the patients concerned to return to be screened on another day.

II) Obviously this sort of approach will be very time-consuming if done with any intention of finding all the high-risk groups in the practice. On top of taking their blood pressure and weight, writing out a form for a cholesterol test takes time.

And of course, after counselling the patient, you will also be faced with dealing with the problem they actually came to see you about in the first place. Few average appointment lists can cope with the strain. The logical answer must be to have a separate screening clinic.

THE CHD SCREENING CLINIC

A separate clinic does have a lot of advantages: it can be run by the practice nurse who can take charge of getting the patients to come, counselling the patient, taking blood pressures, writing out forms and so on, leaving the GP with more time for problem cases and more difficult diagnostic problems.

Another important plus is that such clinics will attract an extra fee in the government's new contract. An FPC might even be persuaded to provide funding for an extra practice nurse should the practice be able to prove it needed one (obviously this will depend upon the generosity of your FPC). Remember, 70% of a practice nurse's salary is re-imbursed so the employment of a practice nurse, combined with the extra income a clinic will provide can prove very cost-effective.

FPCs will require details of the proposed clinic to be entered into the new annual reports. If a good enough argument can be made, many of the more forward-thinking FPCs will try hard to help with resources.

One obvious drawback is that any such clinics can easily take the patient away from the doctor. It is well known that however competent the nurse, patients still give more weight to what their doctor tells them. Since the ultimate reason for the whole exercise is to get patients to change their habits, it can be counterproductive if the doctor is perceived to be removed from the process. It is important that the GP is seen to be involved in the screening clinic and that they are available to reinforce any message that is not getting across.

Clinic organisation

Some of course would say that this is an argument of perfection. Once established a practice nurse can be perceived as more approachable than the doctor and thus becomes just as effective.

The clinic itself must be organised along the same lines as that of any other clinic in the practice. A separate room should be found, stocked with sphygmomanometer, appropriate literature on diet, cholesterol and so on (patient leaflets can be obtained from many sources – see Appendix III for addresses), and an appointment system organised. One patient every 20 to 30 minutes will give enough time for the nurse to examine the patient and give appropriate counselling. In some practices sheer numbers may impose a shorter consultation time.

Next of course the patients themselves must be contacted. The process of doing this will naturally vary from practice to practice.

Since what we are about is primarily screening patients for all coronary heart disease risk factors and not initially just for high cholesterol, the only way of sifting through who is at risk and who isn't is to see everyone between the ages of 25 and 65.

This is not at odds with what has been discussed in Chapter 3 since a cholesterol sample will not be taken from every patient, only from those that are subsequently discovered to be at high risk (realistically that may be about 60 per cent of the practice population).

How do we do this? The easiest way is for a letter of invitation to be given by the receptionist to every patient when they attend the surgery. Since some 70 per cent of patients attend the practice each year, this will ensure an orderly introduction to the new service, preventing any initial rush and at the same time saving postage costs. One idea is to send the invitation out on their birthday thus underlining the fact that the practice cares!

Another alternative is to work steadily through the age–sex register of those patients aged 25 to 60 sending a letter of invitation out in staggered waves over the year.

Lastly the new contract dictates that a GP offer a health check both to all new patients and to any patient who has not been seen for three years. Both of these consultations, probably again best performed by the practice nurse, can be used to check for cholesterol and other CHD risk factors.

Eventually the whole population of the practice will have been screened and all high-risk patients will have had their cholesterol measured (this may take many years). The screening clinic will then continue to screen patients every five years. It is to be hoped that by this time a significant proportion of the practice will be motivated enough to make their own appointments.

It is estimated that if screening such as is described above takes place in an average group practice of 10,000 patients the following will be detected in the 25 to 60 age group:

Patients with a cholesterol > 5.2 mmol/L	6000
Patients with a cholesterol > 7.5 mmol/L	200
Patients with familial hypercholesterolaemia	20
Patients with some other form of familial hyperlipidaemia	25

(For comparison, a 10,000 practice will contain about 200 patients with hypertension.)

Assuming a good uptake from the invitations sent out by the practice it can be assumed that approximately one eighth of the practice population will be screened each year. This will cost the Region about £100,000 per year at 1989 prices – roughly equivalent to three heart transplants or ten coronary artery bypass grafts.

Records

It is imperative that adequate records be kept of all that happens in the screening clinics – separate record cards, summarising what has been discovered in the consultation, must be kept with the notes. Different coloured flags can also be attached to the notes to indicate to the receptionist, doctor or practice nurse that that patient has been screened. If no flag is on view then it will be a signal for the receptionist to arrange an appointment.

Obviously this sort of record is ideally suited to computerisation and as the new contract and the other changes in the White Paper have their effect then it becomes more and more difficult for a practice to exist without one.

The possession of a computer and entry of data into it (again by the practice nurse) means that graphs and statistics can easily be constructed allowing the GP to see quickly and easily the scale of problem and, more importantly, the results of their efforts.

This sort of feedback is of huge importance to any large undertaking since without it the morale of those taking part can easily start to flag.

Finally it goes without saying that records must now be kept in order for the new annual report to be completed.

CHILDREN AND THE ELDERLY

There is no real consensus about what should be done about children. Generally, under the age of 25, young adults and children are less likely to have risk factors such as obesity and hypertension and furthermore many of the features of the various inherited hyperlipidaemias do not manifest themselves until later in life (see Chapter 7).

Table 2. Lipid levels in children – mean (5th, 95th centile)

Age	Total cholesterol (mmol/L)	HDL cholesterol (mmol/L)	Triglyceride (mmol/L)
Newborn	1.8	0.9	0.4
(cord blood)	(1.1–2.1)	(0.3–1.5)	(0.1–0.9)
6 months	3.4	1.3	1.0
	(2.3–4.9)	(0.6–2.2)	(0.6–1.9)
1 year	3.9	1.3	0.9
	(2.5–4.9)	(0.6–2.2)	(0.5–1.8)
2–14 years	4.1	1.7	0.7
	(3.3–5.4)	(0.8–2.6)	(0.4–1.4)

A large GP study of cholesterol screening in children started in the North of England late in 1989 and the results will hopefully provide a good deal of epidemiological data about the prevalence of hypercholesterolaemia in children whether familial or not (Table 2).

At present we do know that at least one in 500 children is born with familial hypercholesterolaemia and that not all of it is picked up; however there are experts who doubt whether cholesterol levels in children provide a real indication of levels in later life.

In general, the best advice for the interested GP is to measure the cholesterol only in children with a positive family history of premature heart disease or hyperlipidaemia.

As for the elderly, the average cholesterol level creeps up with age, though it appears to be more important to control hypertension than to modify cholesterol levels. Unlike hypertension, no really large trials have been carried out to look at the effects of cholesterol on the morbidity and mortality in this age group. All the same it is sensible not to measure the cholesterol in patients over the age of 75.

5
Investigating individual patients

This chapter contains information on the following:

- Protocol for GP investigation of CHD risk
- Pro's and con's of desktop analysers
- Guidelines for analyser use
- Cholesterol results and their interpretation

Now you have your patient in the surgery – what are you going to do with him?

There is much debate about the exact protocol that should be followed in general practice. Certainly it is something that should be discussed among the partners since this is quite an opportunity to find out all manner of things about your patients. If you have an interest now is the time to develop it.

If we stick just to CHD then a useful protocol has recently been suggested by the influential Coronary Prevention Group, an independent team of experts which provides advice in every aspect of CHD prevention.

The CPG suggest GPs follow a three-stage process:

Stage one

- Record the family history, smoking, height, weight, blood pressure and diet (all this can be taken from your patient questionnaire – see Chapter 4).
- Give lifestyle advice and consider drugs for those with persistently raised blood pressure not responding to weight reduction and drinking advice.

Stage two

- Measure cholesterol in the high-risk groups (as described in Chapter 4).
- Give those with raised cholesterol detailed dietary advice.

Stage three

– Screen cholesterol levels throughout the rest of the practice population.

In other words work up the patients in terms of their general CHD risk factors, take cholesterol levels only from those found to be at high risk, then gradually start taking cholesterol levels from the rest of the practice population as time allows.

HOW TO TEST A PATIENT'S BLOOD CHOLESTEROL LEVEL

Testing can be carried out at the hospital pathology laboratory or, if the practice owns a desktop diagnostic device such as a Reflotron, it can be tested by means of a finger-prick at the surgery.

In both instances only the non-fasting total blood cholesterol need be measured initially since this is an accurate enough measure for overall risk (in fact a number of studies have shown it to be by far the most significant lipid risk factor when compared with both HDL cholesterol and triglycerides).

It is best to remember that cholesterol levels should not be measured for three months after a major illness or surgical operation as the serum cholesterol levels will be unusually low. Similarly unrepresentative cholesterol concentrations may be found for up to two weeks after a minor febrile illness or during a period of weight loss.

There has been a good deal of debate over the use of desktop blood analysers outside of hospitals to assess cholesterol levels. Some studies have shown that when used in general practice there can be as much as 1 mmol per litre difference between the GP's reading and those of a hospital laboratory.

The researchers who carried out the famous Helsinki Heart Study (see Appendix II) were for instance convinced that Reflotrons became inaccurate after about six months of use.

Three surveys carried out by a Birmingham team however have shown fairly clearly that these desktop machines used by trained laboratory staff are just as accurate as the more expensive laboratory equipment. They have therefore concluded that poor technique and the use of outdated reagent strips are the main source of inaccuracy in general practice.

GUIDELINES FOR USE OF DESKTOP ANALYSERS (Figure 5)

The group from the Wolfson Research Laboratories at the Department of Clinical Chemistry in Birmingham have published the following helpful guidelines for all GP users of desk top analysers:

1. Before starting any cholesterol measurements contact the head of the clinical chemistry department in your local district general hospital who may be able to advise on selection of equipment and help with training of staff and regular quality control. Ask whether he or she can provide a back-up service for dealing with patients found to have raised cholesterol concentrations.

   If you expect to do fewer than half a dozen cholesterol assays a week it is unlikely that your results will be consistently reliable or the effort worthwhile. It might be better to send the specimens to a recognised laboratory.

2. Make sure that the instrument is installed according to the manufacturer's instructions on a stable flat surface with an adjacent power point. Check on all safety aspects. If the instruction manual has been lost or mislaid request another from the manufacturer.

3. No one should use the instrument unless they have been properly trained, preferably by the manufacturer's representative or staff of the local clinical chemistry department: maintain a list of authorised users. Special quality control specimens (obtainable from the manufacturer) should be analysed repeatedly until everyone is satisfied that the instrument is performing satisfactorily and that the operator is using it correctly. Repeat these tests at regular intervals.

4. All results should be recorded in a note-book or file and kept with the instrument. Record the date, patient's name, age and sex, the result, the batch number of reagents or strips used and the operator's name. Quality control results should be noted here, together with the results of any confirmatory cholesterol assays made on that patient. These records will not only increase the operator's confidence in the results but may be essential evidence if a patient's result is later queried or challenged.

5. Capillary blood specimens should be collected together with proper hygienic technique into heparised tubes (if using a device other than a Reflotron). All contaminated waste material must be disposed of safely. After cleaning the patient's finger with a swab it is essential that any alcohol on the skin is allowed to dry before puncturing the skin and collecting the specimen. Contamination can cause incorrect and misleading results.

6. Check that reagents or strips have not passed their expiry date and discard any that have. Reagents or strips from different batches should not be mixed.

7. The instrument should be cleaned after use and any blood spillages cleaned using a suitable disinfectant, such as 70 per cent isopropanol. Keep the instrument covered when not in use, and maintain it according to the manufacturer's instructions.

35

8. Join an external quality assessment scheme. This is particularly useful in providing an independent check on the performance of your instrument and operator and in showing how they compare with other users.

9. The general practitioner concerned should arrange for all plasma cholesterol results above 6.5 mmol per litre to be confirmed by a recognised laboratory before treatment is started. Similarly, the effect of treatment should be monitored by regular cholesterol assays made by the same hospital laboratory.

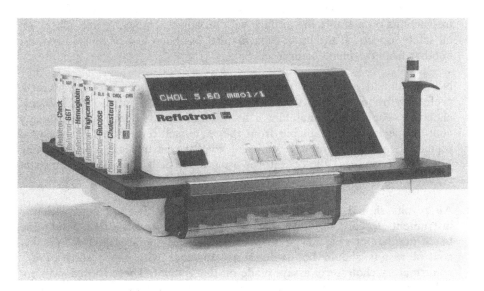

Figure 5. The Reflotron dry chemistry analyser (courtesy of Boehringer–Mannheim UK)

PRO'S AND CON'S OF YOUR OWN ANALYSER

To be honest having your own cholesterol equipment is expensive – a Reflotron at 1989 prices costs £3650 and each test costs £1; thus you've got to be pretty keen and have a lot of patients to have one. The Centre for Health Economics at York University has recently concluded that for most GPs these machines are just too expensive.

They do, however, have the advantage of giving you a result straight away without having to bring the patient back for the result. The drama of having a finger-prick test and getting the result and explanation of the result all at the same time may be more effective at impressing the patient and thus getting them

36

to change their habits, than seeing the doctor and then going off to the hospital laboratory only to return with the results days, maybe weeks later.

Fund holding practices could well be at an advantage if they bought one (although it all rather depends on how much the local laboratory decides to charge for cholesterol testing). Practices that do a lot of occupational health work could also fund these machines on a private basis.

INTERPRETATION OF THE RESULTS

Less than 5.2 mmol per litre: Essentially this is a 'normal' result and the patient can thus be reassured (see Chapter 6 for details). Attention should however still be given to any other abnormal risk factors.

5.2 to 6.5 mmol per litre: The patient should be told that their cholesterol value is a little higher than is desirable, but typical for people in the UK. Correct other risk factors and reassess the cholesterol level in six months.

Levels above 6.5 mmol per litre: Above this level, the amount of triglyceride and HDL cholesterol become important in determining therapy. Since triglyceride levels vary considerably with diet, a fasting (ideally 14 hours) blood sample must be taken and a request made for fasting cholesterol, triglyceride and HDL cholesterol levels made.

As a generalisation cholesterol levels above 5.2 mmol per litre merit some form of treatment (usually dietary).

Triglyceride levels above 5.6 mmol per litre are considered to confer an increased risk of thrombosis although triglyceride has not been shown to be involved in the formation of atherosclerotic plaques (see Appendix I). Levels above 11.0 mmol per litre are associated with an increased risk of pancreatitis.

Levels of HDL cholesterol below 0.9 mmol per litre are linked strongly with the development of CHD particularly if triglyceride levels are above 2.3 mmol per litre.

Occasionally marginally raised levels of cholesterol are due entirely to high levels of HDL in which case the patient can be reassured.

Secondary causes of hyperlipidaemia (see Chapter 9) should also now be excluded by means of a biochemical profile and urinalysis. The profile must include tests for creatinine, urea, transaminases and fasting glucose. Urinalysis must include tests for glucose and protein. Occasionally serum thyroid function tests and immunoglobulins also will be required providing there is adequate clinical suspicion.

The precise interpretation of levels of total serum cholesterol, HDL cholesterol and triglyceride is given in the following chapter. (If you are not altogether clear what HDL cholesterol is, turn to Appendix I for an explanation.)

6
Management in general practice

This chapter contains information on the following:

Introduction

- The problems facing GPs in managing high cholesterol
- An overview of the European Atherosclerosis Society's guidelines
- Basic principles of treatment

Dietary management

- Control of overweight
- Saturated fat reduction
- Exercise
- Increase in fibre
- Practical dietary advice
- Diets in children
- Diet sheet

INTRODUCTION

There is (and probably will continue to be) much debate as to how high levels of blood cholesterol should be managed. To be honest, like so much else in medicine, there is probably no 'right' way – one group of experts will say one thing while another will contradict them. With time, however there will no doubt be a consensus, certainly within countries if not world-wide.

What follows is based on one such consensus – the guidelines published by the European Atherosclerosis Society in 1988. These guidelines have been criticised by many for being, among other things, too rigid and ruled too much by numbers. But although it certainly has its faults these guidelines are, to date, the most workable set of rules that have been produced on a very difficult subject, and without doubt they form a basis on which a GP can work.

MANAGEMENT PROBLEMS IN GENERAL PRACTICE

Before stating exactly what the EAS has said it might be useful at this point just to go over some of the problems facing the GP wanting to treat high cholesterol.

Perhaps the main problem is the patients themselves. As is the case with that other major CHD risk factor, hypertension, the patient looks and feels perfectly normal, even with very high levels of cholesterol. Anything the doctor does by way of treatment that threatens to alter this state of affairs will obviously be resisted particularly if it is proposed that a life-long change of habits takes place.

Unfortunately, the key to managing high blood cholesterol and indeed all the other risk factors involved in CHD is to get patients to do just that. The whole point of detecting patients with high cholesterol is not just to discover those at most risk but also to impress upon them the need to change both their habits of eating and of exercise. This cannot normally be done without some major upheavals.

The crucial difference between treating high cholesterol and so much else in medicine is that the patient cannot be a passive partner in his or her treatment. They cannot just 'take the tablets' and carrying on as normal. The difficult thing about this sort of management (and one that GPs are not particularly used to getting involved with) is that the patient must be motivated to take a very active part in his or her treatment.

The second major problem facing the GP is to decide exactly what they should do in each case. There are a huge number of variables involved in predicting CHD risk and in each patient any number of these might be present. Unlike in other conditions where a choice is usually made between a small number of management options, the path taken in preventing CHD can be highly complex.

Take for example the problem of deciding on treatment in a patient whose cholesterol level is above 6.5 mmol per litre. Any treatment decision must be based on the exact level of total cholesterol, the triglyceride levels, HDL cholesterol levels and the presence or absence of other CHD risk factors. The balance between these and the doctor's knowledge of the individuals themselves must all be taken into account before treatment is begun.

But don't be downhearted. The management of high blood cholesterol is not simple, that is true, but neither should it be beyond the scope of every GP. The EAS guidelines make things easy by splitting the whole subject up into five nicely manageable chunks – therapeutic groups A to E.

OVERVIEW OF EUROPEAN ATHEROSCLEROSIS SOCIETY'S GUIDELINES

Opposite is an overview of what they suggest, and on the following pages a more detailed review of both dietary and drug management will take place.

	Cholesterol (mmol per litre)	Triglyceride (mmol per litre)
Group A	5.2 to 6.5	<2.3

Treatment Guidelines: Advise on a lipid lowering diet and correct any other abnormal risk factors. Drug treatment is almost never needed. Reassess in six months.

Group B	6.5 to 7.8	<2.3

Treatment Guidelines: Advise on a lipid lowering diet which should be monitored by means of LDL-cholesterol levels. If after several months there is no response then consider additional drug therapy, particularly if other risk factors or CHD is present.

Group C	<5.2	2.3 to 5.6

Treatment Guidelines: Advise on an appropriate diet. Drug therapy for mild hypercholesterolaemia is controversial. Look for and treat any causes of hypertriglyceridaemia – obesity, alcohol abuse and diabetes.

Group D	5.2 to 7.8	2.3 to 5.6

Treatment Guidelines: Advise on lipid lowering diet as in Groups B and C. Correct any causes of hypertriglyceridaemia. If after several months there is no response then consider additional drug therapy, particularly if other risk factors or CHD is present.

Group E	>7.8	>5.6

Treatment Guidelines: Specialist advice may be needed with this group. Dietary measures should be attempted first, but drug therapy is commonly required particularly in younger age groups. Control any other CHD risk factors.

GENERAL MANAGEMENT POINTS COMMON TO ALL PATIENTS

1. Treat all modifiable risk factors for CHD, i.e. smoking, obesity, hypertension, diabetes.

   If one or more of these is discovered then the meaning and implications for CHD should be explained to the patient.

2. Any underlying causes of hyperlipidaemia should be sought and if possible treated. A detailed description of what these are and how they raise the lipid levels is to be found in Chapter 9.

   Causes of secondary hyperlipidaemia include: concommitant drug therapy, e.g. thiazide diuretics, β-blockers, oral contraceptives, cortico-steroids; hypothyroidism; cholestasis; bulaemia; alcohol abuse; renal disorders.

3. The reasons why it is important to manage hyperlipidaemia should be explained to the patient and an attempt made to check how much of what you have said has been understood.

   Information should be given both verbally by either the GP or practice nurse and through printed information. A variety of leaflets are produced free of charge by many organisations including drug companies. Those provided by the Health Education Authority and by the Family Heart Association are particularly good (see Appendix III for addresses).

4. The implications of the specific cholesterol reading obtained for that patient should be explained to the patient and ideally he or she should be able to take the figure away with them after the consultation.

PART I: DIETARY MANAGEMENT

The word 'diet' tends to strike terror into the heart of most GPs. Despite the fact that diet is becoming (and probably always has been) a major tool in the fight against disease and particularly disease prevention, there is precious little taught about it in medical schools.

In many ways this is surprising since it is improvements in diet, linked to better standards of public health that have made such a difference to overall mortality in this country and the rest of the world over the past couple of hundred years. Medical schools are however packed with information about diseases and their treatments, while diet somehow gets thrust to one side.

This gap in medical education obviously hasn't caused too many problems in the past however. GPs have always got by, handing out a diet sheet when they can, and offering encouragement and advice to erstwhile slimmers when the need arises. But really it needn't necessarily be so.

It is of course possible to offload all advice on diet to the practice nurse or to a dietician if you can get one to see your patient. But clearly it would be nicer if you too had the information at your finger tips.

What follows is a beginners guide to the dietary management of hyperlipidaemias.

National dietary guidelines

Since the beginning of the 1980s several major reports on nutrition have emphasised the need for the British public to change their eating habits. The two most important were those produced by the National Advisory Committee on Nutrition Education (NACNE) and the Committee on Medical Aspects of Food Policy (COMA). Although there were some differences in their precise recommendations, the principles they have put forward form the basis for this country's diet policy. They include lowering the total fat intake, raising slightly the intake of polyunsaturated fat and lowering the intake of saturated fats and finally increasing the fibre intake (Figure 6).

The diet endorsed by both NACNE and COMA for the general population is more or less appropriate for the majority of patients with hyperlipidaemia. Let's look in more detail at the broad goals of this diet.

1. to control weight
2. to reduce the intake of saturated fats to 10 per cent or less of the total number of calories in the diet
3. to replace partially saturated fats with mono- and polyunsaturated fats
4. to reduce dietary cholesterol to 300 mg or less per day
5. to increase consumption of soluble fibre

Overall the total amount of fat in the food should be reduced from what can in some circumstances be as high as 50 per cent (especially if a lot of processed and 'junk' food are consumed) to about 30 (NACNE) or 35 per cent (COMA) of the diet.

It is calculated that if these fat levels are achieved then the average blood cholesterol level in this country will fall from about 5.9 mmol per litre to perhaps 5.0 mmol per litre.

N.B. In the USA a much lower target level of fat has been set, which would bring the average level of cholesterol down to about 4.8 mmol per litre.

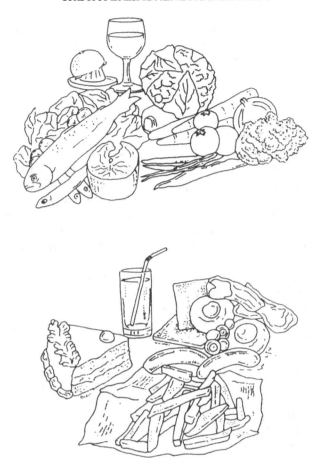

Figure 6. Good and bad foods

Controlling the weight

Weight control is one of the most effective means of reducing elevated lipid levels, yet oddly this step is usually omitted in treatment.

Patients should be encouraged to reach their ideal body weight. This can be ascertained either from looking at standard height weight charts (Table 3) (which tend to be pretty unreliable) or by calculating the patient's body mass index – this should ideally be at a level of between 20 and 25:

$$\text{Body mass index} = \text{weight (kg)}/(\text{height in m})^2$$

Naturally, there will be many patients who are already at an ideal weight. These people should not be recommended to lose more weight. A low-fat diet, not a weight reducing diet should be recommended.

The rest however, will need both diets.

Recommending a certain calorie diet – say an 800 or 1000 calories a day diet – although theoretically correct, is a waste of time for most patients. Faced with a portion of food and no packet, or having to eat part and not all of a packet of food, can make any calculation the patient may wish to make almost impossible.

Table 3. Guidelines for body weight. The minimum level for diagnosing obesity is taken as 20% above the upper limit of the acceptable weight range

Height without shoes (m)	Men Weight without clothes (kg)			Women Weight without clothes (kg)		
	Average	Acceptable weight range	Obese	Average	Acceptable weight range	Obese
1.45				46.0	42–53	64
1.48				46.5	42–54	65
1.50				47.0	43–55	66
1.52				48.5	44–57	68
1.54				49.5	44–58	70
1.56				50.4	45–58	70
1.58	55.8	51–64	77	51.3	46–59	71
1.60	57.6	52–65	78	52.6	48–61	73
1.62	58.6	53–66	79	54.0	49–62	74
1.64	59.6	54–67	80	55.4	50–64	77
1.66	60.6	55–69	83	56.8	51–63	78
1.68	61.7	56–71	85	58.1	52–66	79
1.70	63.5	58–73	88	60.0	53–67	80
1.72	65.0	59–74	89	61.3	55–69	83
1.74	66.5	60–75	90	62.6	56–70	84
1.76	68.0	62–77	92	64.0	58–72	86
1.78	69.4	64–79	95	65.3	59–74	89
1.80	71.0	65–80	96			
1.82	72.6	66–82	98			
1.84	74.2	67–84	101			
1.86	75.8	69–86	103			
1.88	77.6	71–88	106			
1.90	79.3	73–90	108			
1.92	81.0	75–93	112			
BMI	22.0	20.1–25.0	30.0	20.8	18.7–23.8	28.6

It is better just to advise changing from inappropriate to appropriate foods and to encourage the patient not to overeat. Reassure the patient that a weight loss of as little as 2 kg per month is perfectly satisfactory and set intermediate target weights to prevent them becoming disillusioned.

Realistically, few patients can be expected to achieve the overall change in their diet within a period of less than several months; thus it is important for the GP or practice nurse to book the patient in for regular weight measurements and advice sessions.

If a patient continues to put on weight or does not achieve a satisfactory fall, it may be useful for a patient to join with others in fighting the flab. A number of organisations, most notably Weight Watchers, organise group sessions in most areas, where peer group pressure can be brought to bear on the subject. This method is particularly useful for mothers who are having to cook meals for the rest of the (non-dieting) family.

Nutri System, a highly successful US slimming company is currently opening a number of its centres up and down the UK. Their system involves both dietary advice and much-needed counselling. Patients pay a flat fee (half of which is returned if they stick with the system for 12 months) but must, initially at least, purchase all their foodstuffs from Nutri System itself. The system is proving both effective and popular.

Finally it must be impressed upon these patients that this dieting will be life-long, not just a one-off. Many patients work hard to lose a few pounds, then go straight back to eating as they used to as soon as their target has been reached. A positive outlook on weight and dieting should be encouraged.

Actually advising the patient

Ideally a GP need only refer these patients to a community dietician and his or her problems would be over. However, due to the extreme lack of these skilled individuals, it is unusual for a GP to be able to make use of this resource.

GPs and practice nurses are not dieticians, nor should they be; however there are a number of basic rules to follow and a number of tips to pick up when trying to deal with dietary problems in general practice.

First, before making any plans as to what a patient should and should not be eating in the future, the GP/nurse must take a simple dietary history to establish exactly what the patient is eating at present.

Perhaps the easiest way to do this is to ask the patient about what he or she eats in an average day. For example:

7.00 am   Branflakes, toast, tea
10.00 am Sandwich (egg and bacon), tea
12.00   More sandwiches, cake, tea
3.00 pm   Tea, biscuits

6.00 pm   Meat (roast, sausages, chop)
           Potatoes (chips)
           Vegetables
           Pie and custard/ice cream
10.00 pm   Milk drink
Four pints of beer at the weekend

Next the patient should be weighed and their desirable weight (not necessarily the average weight for their height) worked out.

Armed with these findings, the GP/nurse can then start to advise the patient specifically as to what should be restricted and what maintained; whether the patient needs to lose weight and so on. They should be encouraged to learn more about the food they eat.

For most people the provision of a simple diet sheet (Table 4) and some recipes, together with some general advice about eating will now be all that is needed. The patient should be brought back to the surgery at regular intervals to check on weight gain or loss and for encouragement to stick to the diet.

Sticking to the diet can of course be the hardest part, particularly for working class families where knowledge about food is sparse and the pressure not to find alternatives to the fried fatty food that most of this country eats is hardest to resist. The problems of weening some of these patients off the diet they have been used to, then putting them onto a lipid lowering regime, should not be underestimated.

Another major problem for patients coming from poorer, working class backgrounds is cost. Many patients see dieting as something that needs special expensive foods and is thus impossible for them even to consider. In reality, however, a lipid lowering diet is usually much cheaper than a normal Western diet, since there are fewer expensive packaged and processed foods and less red meat. This should be explained to the patient.

Children

Managing high blood cholesterol is not easy in children. A similar diet to that for adults can be recommended for children, but it can be very difficult to make them comply with it (and even more difficult to make sure they comply with it outside of the home – at school or at play).

Exercise

Exercise is an essential part of the dieting process. But its main benefit is not in helping to lose calories (although any increase in energy expenditure will help to burn up a few calories); more important is the psychological benefit that exercise brings.

Table 4. Dietary advice for patients with hyperlipidaemia

	Recommended	Eat in moderation	Foods to avoid
Cereals	wholemeal flour; oatmeal; wholemeal or granary bread; wholegrain cereals; porridge oats; crispbreads; wholegrain rice and pasta	white flour; white bread; sugar-coated breakfast cereals; white rice and pasta	fancy breads, e.g. croissants, savoury cheese biscuits, cream crackers
Fruit and vegetables	all fresh and frozen vegetables, e.g. peas, broad beans, sweetcorn; pulses, e.g. kidney beans, lentils; potatoes (boiled or jacket – eat skins wherever possible); fresh fruit; dried fruit; tinned fruit in natural juice	chips and roast potatoes if cooked in suitable oil or fat; avocado pears	potato crisps and savoury snacks, chips cooked in unsuitable oil or fat
Nuts	walnuts	almonds, Brazil nuts, chestnuts, hazelnuts, peanuts	coconut
Fish	all fresh or frozen white and oily, e.g. herrings, tuna, cod, plaice; tinned fish in tomato sauce or brine, e.g. sardines, pilchards	shellfish occasionally	fish roe
Meat	lean white meats, e.g. chicken, turkey veal, rabbit, game	not more than three times a week: lean meats, e.g. ham, beef, pork, lamb, bacon lean mince; occasionally offal, e.g. liver, kidney	visible fat on meat (including crackling), sausages, pâté, duck, goose, streaky bacon, faggots, meat pies, meat pasties

(continued)

48

	Recommended	Eat in moderation	Foods to avoid
Eggs and dairy produce	skimmed milk, skimmed milk cheese, e.g. cottage and curd cheese, Quark; egg white (3 egg yolks per week only)	semi-skimmed milk; Edam, Camembert, Parmesan, Mozzarella	whole milk; cream; hard cheese, e.g. Cheshire, Cheddar and Stilton; cream cheese; desserts made with full cream milk; excess egg yolks (more than 3 per week); mayonnaise
Fats	all fats should be limited	margarine labelled 'high in polyunsaturates'; corn oil; sunflower oil; soya oil; safflower oil	butter, dripping, suet lard, margarine not labelled 'high in polyunsaturates'; cooking/vegetable oil of unknown origin; palm oil, coconut oil
Puddings, desserts, cakes and biscuits	skimmed milk puddings; low-fat puddings, e.g. jelly, sorbet, low-fat yoghurts; skimmed milk sauces; pastry puddings, crumbles, cakes and biscuits made with suitable margarine or oil and wholemeal flour	pastry, puddings, cakes and biscuits made with suitable margarine or oil and white flour; ice cream	tinned or whole milk puddings; dairy ice cream; pastry, puddings, crumbles, cakes, biscuits and sauces made with whole milk, eggs or unsuitable fat or oil; chocolate or cream-filled biscuits or cakes; all proprietary puddings and sauces
Sweets, preserves and spreads	Bovril, Oxo, Marmite; low-sugar jams and marmalades	meat and fish pastes; boiled sweets, fruit pastilles, peppermints, etc.; jam, marmalade, honey, sugar; high-fibre snackbars made with fruit, nuts and whole grains	peanut butter, chocolate, toffees, fudge, butterscotch, lemon curd, mincemeat; chocolate or cream-filled sweets and confectionary
Drinks	tea, coffee (made with skimmed milk); mineral water; unsweetened fruit juices; clear soups, homemade soups, e.g. vegetable, lentils, etc.	packet soups, alcohol	cream soups

49

Three or four 20-minute sessions a week spent doing aerobic exercise such as walking briskly, jogging, swimming, cycling (depending on the age and fitness of the individual) rapidly makes the patient feel better since it improves cardiovascular function and acts as a catalyst, awakening them to the benefits of being healthy and reviving both esteem and self-control. Most clinics find that getting patients to stick to a diet is far more difficult without exercise.

All patients should be advised to gradually build up their exercise programme rather than jumping in from the outset with very heavy exercise.

One last benefit of exercise is that it appears to increase HDL levels.

Reduction in saturated fats and increase in mono- and polyunsaturates

It is not unusual to find individuals consuming as much as 40 or even 50 per cent of their total energy requirement each day as fat. Often much of this is saturated animal fats. As has already been discussed the overall total must be reduced to at least 30 per cent, no more than one third of which should be saturated.

That means cutting down on most red meat (which supplies about a quarter of the total saturated fats consumed), butter and margarine (another quarter) full cream milk and cheese (another quarter) and cooking fats, chocolate, pastries and the like (which contain an awful lot of hidden saturated fat).

A useful rule of thumb is to allow red meat to be eaten no more than three times a week.

Obviously it is not feasible to cut out fats completely; thus some of the reduction in saturated fats can be replaced by both polyunsaturated fats such as soft margarines and by monosaturated fats – olive oil.

Oily fish (such as tuna) in particular seems to be valuable in reducing CHD risk since it contains a lot of polyunsaturated fats. Eskimos and other fish eating nations like the Japanese have very low levels of CHD and much has been made of the protective effect conferred by fish on these people.

The consumption of fish oil seems to be particularly effective at reducing triglyceride levels.

Nations who eat a lot of monounsaturated oils, such as the peoples of the Mediterranean, also have a low incidence of CHD. The typical Italian diet for instance is not only rich in monounsaturates, it also contains a lot of soluble fibre (see below) which seems to add to the protective effect.

No specific reduction of dietary cholesterol per se is usually needed. If the total fat intake is restricted then the cholesterol levels is usually reduced with it anyway.

The ideal is 300 mg per day. Cholesterol is contained principally in eggs, dairy products and shellfish.

Increase in the amount of soluble fibre in the diet

The main compensation for the reduction in fat in the diet must be an increase in the amount of carbohydrate. Since fat is a major energy source something must replace it. So eat more pasta and baked potatoes – but don't eat too much (and don't put butter on them!).

Most experts recommend eating about 30 g of fibre a day (most people in the UK eat about 20 g) both as the insoluble form such as bran, and the soluble form – cooked dried beans, lentils, fruit and oats.

Insoluble fibre acts by absorbing water to improve bowel functioning and protecting against diverticulitis, haemorrhoids and even bowel cancer.

Soluble fibre probably acts by binding bile cholesterol in the entero hepatic circulation preventing it from being reabsorbed. Oats and beans have been particularly singled out of late as a useful lipid lowerer.

In general every attempt should be made to eat unprocessed rather than processed carbohydrates since much of the lipid lowering abilities of the carbohydrate disappear in the latter. This means eating more wholemeal bread, more fresh vegetables and so on.

In patients with hypertriglyceridaemia, all forms of sugar should be massively reduced since these can exacerbate the conditions.

Alcohol

A modest amount of alcohol is probably quite good for you, but too much particularly if the triglyceride levels are high, should be discouraged. 12 units a week is a maximum (less in women). It should also not be forgotten that alcohol is a major source of calories.

In summary

Fat: less than 30 per cent of energy intake – reduce saturated fats and partially replace with poly- and monounsaturates

Carbohydrate: 50 to 60 per cent – mainly unprocessed full-fibre products (soluble fibre)

Protein: 10 to 15 per cent – mainly vegetable protein

Cholesterol: – less than 300 mg per day

All in all, for most people who eat a normal Western diet, the adoption of a lipid lowering diet will reduce their blood cholesterol by about 20 per cent. This will be even greater if this diet is combined with weight loss although the GP or whoever is advising the patient should remember that weight loss is not desirable in every patient. Once the desired weight has been achieved, every effort should be made to reduce the lipid levels while keeping the actual energy intake constant.

A maximal reduction in lipid levels can take several months to achieve because of the need for repeated instruction and encouragement. In some cases the desired level of blood cholesterol is never reached and at that stage a careful study of a patient's compliance with the diet and a consideration of a more stringent diet must be made.

7
Drug management

This chapter contains information on the following:

- Patients likely to need drug therapy
- Bile acid resins
- Fibrates
- Nicotinic acid derivatives
- HMG CoA reductase inhibitors
- Fish oils

INTRODUCTION

It cannot be emphasised too strongly that diet, not drugs, is the mainstay of treatment in all forms of hyperlipidaemia. Only after a prolonged effort to reduce the levels of cholesterol and triglyceride has been made, and the patient's compliance checked and double-checked, should drugs be considered. In practice this may mean trying dietary measures for as long as 10 months.

In reality the final decision can only be made after weighing up the risks and benefits of treatment in that individual. Age, the presence or absence of heart disease, and of course the level of cholesterol or triglyceride, must obviously all be taken into account.

PATIENTS MORE LIKELY TO NEED DRUGS

In general the following patients are usually treated with drugs earlier rather than later:

- those with a primary hyperlipidaemic syndrome especially familial hyper-cholesterolaemia, familial combined hypercholesterolaemia and remnant particle disease (see Chapter 9).

- a young male patient with a strong family history of CHD

- patients with pre-existing CHD and total cholesterol >6.5 mmol/L

- patients at high risk of developing CHD (e.g. diabetic or hypertensive) with total cholesterol levels greater than 7.8 mmol/L

- a patient with hypertriglyceridaemia at risk of pancreatitis

Naturally, if a patient is started on lipid lowering drugs then they must remain on a strict lipid lowering diet. All other CHD risk factors must also be controlled.

Some experts recommend that hospital consultants not GPs start patients on lipid lowering drugs. There is no reason this should be, providing the GP has a good knowledge of the drugs he or she is using and the conditions in which they should be used.

In truth the drug treatment of hyperlipidaemia can seem a bit confusing. There are a number of effective drugs on the market, yet it is certainly not correct to believe that each of them could be suitable for your patient. They have their own properties and side-effects and each should therefore be used in a precise manner.

To bring some form of simplification into their classification, lipid lowering drugs can be split into two groups: those that lower cholesterol levels alone, and those that lower both cholesterol and triglyceride levels.

(Study Appendix I before reading further if your knowledge of lipid metabolism is not good.)

DRUGS THAT LOWER SERUM CHOLESTEROL ALONE

Bile acid exchange resins: cholestyramine (Figure 7) and colestipol

These are very much first line therapy in patients with very high levels of serum cholesterol. Using these drugs reductions of up to 30 per cent in LDL cholesterol can be achieved; HDL is usually raised slightly. Triglycerides may however also rise a little so these drugs should not be used alone in patients whose triglyceride is high.

Both cholestyramine and colestipol have been shown to be particularly useful in reducing CHD morbidity and mortality if used in combination with other drugs. Studies have shown them to be effective if combined with either nicotonic acid or an HMGCoA reductase inhibitor. Such combinations have been shown to lead to atheroma regression in patients with pre-existing CHD.

Mechanism of action: They bind with bile salts in the gut and prevent them from being reabsorbed. This means that the liver then has to produce more bile salts and this begins to use up the available cholesterol. As a result more LDL receptors in the liver become free leading to an increase in LDL catabolism.

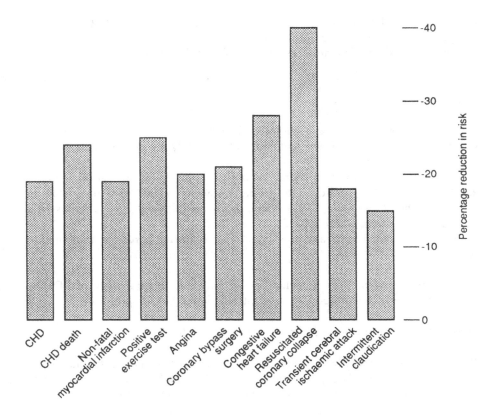

Figure 7. The effect of cholestyramine on coronary morbidity. Patients treated with cholestyramine in the Lipid Research Clinics Trial had a 15 to 40 per cent reduction in coronary morbidity compared with those patients who were treated with placebo

Dose: Cholestyramine (Questran) – 12 to 24 g daily in divided doses (one sachet = 4 g). Start with a dose of one sachet three times a day, half an hour before meals. Slowly increase as required. Both available formulations of cholestyramine are orange-flavoured, to mask the unpleasant amine taste.

Colestipol (Colestid) – 5 to 30 g daily in one or two divided doses. Sachets should be dispersed in an appropriate amount of liquid and shaken. Since the powder resin can taste gritty, but is tasteless, many patients add it to breakfast cereal, muesli, porridge or yoghurt, which successfully disguises the texture.

Side-effects: Constipation, nausea and bloating are the main side-effects, and tend to be dosage related, although more rarely colicky pains and diarrhoea may be complained of. Since they may affect the absorption of other drugs, these are best taken about one hour beforehand.

Children and lactating mothers will need folic acid supplements.

Probucol

Probucol is not as effective a cholesterol lowerer as the bile sequestrants. It reduces LDL by up to 15 per cent, but unfortunately it can also reduce HDL, thus limiting its usefulness.

Probucol does however seem to possess the ability to shrink tendon xanthomata. It has anti-oxidant properties which could give it a role in preventing the development of atheroma. If proven, this property could make it a very useful drug in preventing CHD.

Probucol is used generally only in patients requiring agressive combination therapy.

Mechanism of action: This is unclear, but it may lead to catabolism of LDL by being somehow incorporated into the central lipid core of lipoproteins.

Dose: Probucol (Lurselle) – 500 mg twice daily with food.

Side-effects: It is generally well tolerated, but may occasionally cause nausea and flatulance. Occasionally a prolongation of the QT interval can occur on ECG making it advisable not to give it to patients with ischaemic heart disease.

DRUGS THAT LOWER BOTH CHOLESTEROL AND TRIGLYCERIDE

Fibric acid derivatives: clofibrate, bezafibrate, fenofibrate and gemfibrozil

These drugs lower the levels of both cholesterol and triglyceride by reducing the concentration of VLDL. This can lead to a lowering of LDL and in the process increases HDL. They can be regarded as 'broad spectrum' lipid lowerers. Fibrates are used mainly in the treatment of mixed hyperlipidaemia (type IIB) when both cholesterol and triglyceride are raised.

Gemfibrozil was used with good effect in the Helsinki Heart trial. There is not a lot to choose between these drugs in terms of efficacy – side-effects and cost are the main determinants.

These drugs can be used in combination with the bile acid resins if the level of cholesterol proves difficult to control using one alone.

Mode of action: There is an increase in the activity of the enzyme lipoprotein lipase leading to an increase in the breakdown of triglyceride. Fibrates may also reduce cholesterol synthesis through a non-specific inhibition of HMGCoA reductase.

Dose: Clofibrate (Atromid-S) – 500 mg 2 to 3 times daily after meals.
Bezafibrate (Bezalip, Bezalip-Mono) – 200 mg tds with or after meals / 200 mg bd in hypertriglyceridaemia.
Fenofibrate (Lipantil) – 300 mg daily in divided doses with food.
Gemfibrozil (Lopid) – 1.2 g daily in two divided doses (range 0.9 to 1.5 g daily).

Side-effects: The incidence of side-effects with the last three drugs in the list is low (they are often used if a bile acid resin has to be withdrawn because of side effects). GI upsets, a reversible myopathy and impotence may rarely occur. Renal failure is a contraindication for therapy. In patients with hypertriglyceridaemia, they may increase the total and LDL cholesterol.

Clofibrate, the first drug of this class, has been shown to increase the excretion of cholesterol in the bile and thus increases the incidence of gall stones. An early WHO trial also showed an increase in deaths from all causes other than myocardial infarction.

Nicotinic acid derivatives: nicotinic acid, nicofuranose, acipimox

The nicotinic acid derivatives are potentially very effective drugs at reducing both cholesterol and triglyceride, but their level of side-effects is such that at truly therapeutic doses a large proportion of patients have to stop taking them. Newer drugs, such as acipimox, may have reduced this problem.
Again these drugs can be used effectively if combined with resins in cases of severe familial hypercholesterolaemia. They should be used with caution however if combined with a HMGCoA inhibitor since there seems to be an increased risk of myopathy.

Mode of action: They have a number of effects including inhibiting the release of fatty acids from adipose tissue, thus reducing the flow of these particles to the liver for the synthesis of lipoproteins. They also probably inhibit lipoprotein lipase.

Dose: Nicotinic acid – 100 to 200 mg tds gradually increased over two to four weeks to 1–2 g daily.
Nicofuranose (Bradilan) – 0.5 to 1.0 g tds.
Acipimox (Olbetam) – 500 to 750 g daily in divided doses.

Side-effects: Flushing is the main side-effect. This can be reduced by starting at a low dose given with meals and concurrently giving the patient an aspirin. Unfortunately the drug is often only effective at high doses when side-effects become intolerable.

Other side-effects include gout and a rise in liver enzymes. They should not be given if the patient has a peptic ulcer.

HMG-CoA reductase inhibitors: simvastatin and pravastatin

These drugs are remarkably effective in reducing LDL as well as in reducing triglyceride and increasing HDL cholesterol. LDL reductions of up to 30 per cent have been recorded and up to 70 per cent if given in combination with a resin.

Simvastatin and pravastatin are the first in a long line of new HMGCoA reductase inhibitors currently in development. At the time of going to press only two are available in the UK.

Since these are new drugs their efficacy is still being assessed (all side-effects must be reported to the CSM). Despite their promise they must, for the moment, be regarded as third-line agents.

Mode of action: These drugs act within cells to inhibit HMGCoA reductase, the key enzyme responsible for cholesterol synthesis. By reducing cellular cholesterol synthesis, particularly in the liver, the number of LDL receptors increase and thus lower LDL levels.

Dose: Simvastatin (Zocor) – initially 10 mg nocte, adjusting at minimum four-week intervals according to response to a maximum of 40 mg.
Pravastatin (Lipostat) – initially 10 mg nocte, adjusting at four-week intervals according to response to maximum of 40 mg.

Side-effects: Abnormalities in liver function can occur and at present should be monitored by carrying out tests for LFTs four to six weekly for the first 12 months of treatment, then periodically.

Other side-effects reported include constipation, flatulence, headache, nausea and occasionally a myopathy.

Simvastatin should not be used in combination with warfarin, digoxin, fibrates, nicotinic acid or cyclosporin, and should not normally be given to children, or women of child-bearing age not using an appropriate contraceptive method. Pravastatin has no significant drug interactions, but should also not be given to women of child-bearing age or individuals less than 18 years old.

Other lipid-lowering drugs

Fish oils: Fish oils contain omega-3-fatty acids which are effective in reducing plasma triglycerides but have little effect, except at very high dosage on cholesterol levels.

Maxepa, the only fish oil currently licensed, should only be used to treat severe hypertriglyceridaemia. Dose: five capsules or 5 ml bd with food. Side-effects: nausea and eructation.

Table 5. Profiles of frequently prescribed lipid-lowering drugs (to be used only as adjunctive therapy to a prudent diet)

Characteristics	Probucol	Resins	
		Cholestyramine HCl	Colestipol
Indications*	For reduction of elevated serum cholesterol in patients with primary hypercholesterolaemia (elevated low density lipoproteins) who have not responded adequately to diet, weight reduction, and control of diabetes mellitus. May be useful in combined hypercholesterolaemia and hypertriglyceridaemia, but not where hypertriglyceridaemia is the abnormality of most concern	Adjunctive therapy to diet for the reduction of elevated serum cholesterol in patients with primary hypercholesterolaemia (elevated low density lipoprotein [LDL] cholesterol) who do not respond adequately to diet. May be useful to lower LDL cholesterol in patients who also have hypertriglyceridaemia, but it is not indicated where hypertriglyceridaemia is the abnormality of most concern	Indicated as adjunctive therapy to diet for the reduction of elevated serum cholesterol in patients with primary hypercholesterolaemia (elevated low density lipoproteins). Has been shown to have no effect on or to increase triglyceride levels.
Total cholesterol-reducing efficacy	10.7–27% reduction	13.4–25% reduction	13.4–25% reduction
Most commonly reported adverse reactions*	Most commonly affected is GI tract: diarrhoea, flatulence, abd. pain, nausea, and vomiting	Constipation (occasionally with fecal impaction), abd. pain and distension, belching, flatulence, nausea, vomiting and diarrhoea	Constipation (occasionally with fecal impaction), abdominal discomfort, (abd. pain and distension), flatulence, nausea, vomiting, diarrhoea
Less commonly reported reactions, but worth noting*	Prolongation of QT interval in some patients	Increased bleeding tendency (due to vit. K deficiency) with long-term use – possible hyperchloremic acidosis in children	Increased bleeding tendency from vit. K deficiency, increase in serum triglycerides

THESE PRODUCTS ALSO CAUSE SIDE-EFFECTS AND ADVERSE REACTIONS INVOLVING VARIOUS SYSTEMS IN ADDITION TO THOSE LISTED. PRESCRIBING INFORMATION FOR EACH DRUG SHOULD BE READ CAREFULLY BEFORE IT IS PRESCRIBED

Known interaction with other drug*	The combination of clofibrate and probucol is not recommended – see Prescribing Information	Yes (may bind a variety of other drugs given concomitantly, delaying or reducing their absorption – see Prescribing Information in PDR)	Yes (may delay or reduce absorption of concomitant oral medication, particularly of chlorothiazine, tetracycline and penicillin. May affect availability of digitalis preparations)

* Taken from *Physicians Desk Reference*, 41st edn., Medical Economics Company Inc., Oradell, NJ. 1987 (under each product name).

| cotinic acid | Simvastatin | Fibric acid compounds | |
		Clofibrate	Gemfibrozil
djunctive therapy in tients with significant perlipidaemia (elevated olesterol and/or glycerides) who do not spond adequately to et and weight loss	As an adjunct to diet for the reduction of elevated total and LDL cholesterol levels in patients with primary hypercholest-erolaemia (types IIa and IIb) when the response to diet and other non-pharmacological measures alone has been inadequate	For primary dysbetalipo-proteinaemia (type III hyperlipidaemia) that does not respond adequately to diet. May be considered for the treatment of adult patients with very high (in excess of 750 mg/dl) serum triglyceride levels (types IV and V hyperlipidaemia) who present a risk of abdominal pain and pancreatitis and who do not respond to diet	For the treatment of adult patients with very high (in excess of 750 mg/dl) serum triglyceride levels (types IV or V hyperlipoprotein-aemia) who present a risk of abdominal pain and pancreatitis and who do not respond to a deter-mined dietary effort to control them
		Patients with triglyceride levels in excess of 750 mg/dl are likely to present such risk. Both products have little effect on elevated cholesterol levels in most subjects	
% reduction	18–34% reduction (depending on dosage)	6.5–9% reduction	1.8–8.6% reduction*
vere flushing, activtion peptic ulcers, pertension	Increase in serum transaminase levels, headache, constipation, diarrhoea, dyspepsia, abd. pain and cramping, nausea	Most common is nausea; less frequent GI reactions are vomiting, loose stools, dyspepsia, flatulence and abd. distress	Most frequently reported involve GI system, viz. (in decreasing order of frequency): abd. pain, diarrhoea, nausea, vomiting, flatulence
normal liver function ts, jaundice, GI orders, decreased cose tolerance	Myopathy	Increased incidence of cholelithiasis, flu-like symptoms, increase in cardiac arrhythmias and intermittent claudication, possible increased risk of malignancies	The less commonly reported adverse reactions of clofibrate may also apply to gemfibrozil
s tihypertensive drugs)	Warfarin	Yes (anticoagulants)	Yes (anticoagulants)

8
Specific guidelines for treatment

This chapter contains details on the following:

Practical management based on the European Atherosclerosis Society's guidelines
- The 'normal' patient
- Treatment Group A
- Treatment Group B
- Treatment Group C
- Treatment Group D
- Treatment Group E
- Follow up
- A simpler alternative

Armed with a little knowledge about both diet and drugs, we can now move on to looking specifically at how best to treat individual patients. It cannot be said too often that a decision on treatment must be based not only on the patient's lipid level, but also on the presence or absence of other CHD risk factors. However to make things somewhat easier to understand, we will consider treatment following the therapeutic groups A to E as discussed earlier.

NORMAL (cholesterol < 5.2 mmol per litre)

Despite the fact that a patient's examination and investigations appear normal, the GP or practice nurse should still make as much use as possible of the time they have with that patient.

As was mentioned earlier, if a patient is simply reassured that his cholesterol level and/or blood pressure are OK, then this tends to act as an disincentive when it comes to living a more healthy life. 'Normal' patients often get the impression that everything can now continue to be normal for the rest of their lives no matter what they do.

Every patient must be properly counselled on the various CHD risk factors and the message drummed home by giving some appropriate literature on the subject. Patients dealt with in this way will, it is hoped, continue to try hard to avoid the disease.

Test the cholesterol, blood pressure and so on at five yearly intervals.

GROUP A (cholesterol 5.2 to 6.5 mmol per litre/triglycerides <2.3 mmol per litre)

CHD risk: Twofold increase in risk for patients with cholesterol levels of 6.5 mmol per litre.

Mangement plan:

i)   If no other CHD risk factor present
     Advise on weight control if necessary and discuss lipid lowering diet. There is no need for regular follow-up other than a re-check in about 5 years.

ii) If other risk factors are present

Step I: Again advise on a lipid lowering diet and weight control if necessary. Any associated risk factors should be controlled as appropriate.
↓
Step II: Re-assess in 6 months
If treatment goals have been reached then re-assess in five years. If the desired treatment goals have not been reached then the content of and the patient's compliance with the diet should be reviewed. Always encourage the patient.
↓
Step III: Re-assess in 6 to 12 months
Repeat the above process
↓
Step IV: Re-assess in 12 months
If the desired treatment goals have been achieved re-assess in five years. If the LDL cholesterol is between 3.5 and 4.0 mmol per litre then encourage diet and compliance with it. If the LDL cholesterol is greater than 4.0 mmol per litre despite good compliance with the diet, then very occasionally drug therapy will be needed.

Long term: Re-assess at 3 to 5 yearly intervals if on diet alone. If on diet and drugs then re-assess every 3 months increasing to 12 month intervals.

GROUP B (cholesterol 6.5 to 7.8 mmol per litre/triglyceride <2.3 mmol per litre)

CHD risk: Risk is high and increases steeply.

Management plan:

i) If no other CHD risk factor present
Step I: A lipid lowering diet and weight control should be advised upon. Any underlying causes of one or both should be dealt with.
↓
Step II: Re-assess in 2 to 4 months
If the treatment goal is achieved then re-assess in 12 months. If the treatment goal is not achieved then review the patient's diet and their compliance with it.
↓
Step III: Re-assess in 3 to 6 months
If the treatment goal is achieved then re-assess in 12 months. If the treatment goal is not achieved then review diet and encourage compliance.
↓
Step IV: Re-assess at 3 to 6 months
If treatment goal is achieved then re-assess in 12 months. If the treatment goal is not achieved despite the patient complying well with the diet, then consider drug therapy.

ii) If other risk factors are present

Step I: Control associated risk factors and any underlying causes of raised lipids. Place on lipid lowering diet plus weight reducing diet if necessary.
↓
Step II: Re-assess in 2 to 4 months
If treatment goals achieved then re-assess in 12 months. If treatment goals not achieved then review diet and patient's compliance with it.
↓
Step III: Re-assess in 3 to 6 months
If treatment goal achieved then re-assess in 12 months. If treatment goal not achieved then consider the addition of drug therapy. A fasting lipid profile will be required for HDL, triglyceride and LDL levels.
↓
Step IV: Re-assess in 2 to 4 months
If treatment goal not achieved then consider an increase in drug dosage and encourage dietary compliance.

Long term: Re-assess at 1 to 3 year intervals if on diet alone and at 3 monthly intervals increasing to every year if on diet and drug therapy.

GROUP C (cholesterol <5.2 mmol per litre/triglyceride 2.3 to 5.6 mmol per litre)

CHD risk: controversial, probably fairly low.

Management plan:

Step I: Correct any weight problem and any underlying causes – especially alcohol overindulgence. Advise on lipid lowering diet and control any associated CVD risk factors.
↓
Step II: Re-assess in 6 to 12 months
If treatment goal achieved, then follow-up in 3 to 5 years. If treatment goal not achieved encourage compliance with all measures described in step I.
↓
Step III: Re-assess in 6 to 12 months
As in step I.
↓
Step IV: If treatment goal achieved follow up in 3 to 5 years. If treatment goal not achieved consider referral to specialised centre. Drug treatment for moderate hypertriglyceridaemia is highly controversial.

Long term: Re-assess at 1 to 5 yearly intervals if treated by diet alone and at 3 monthly increasing to one yearly if on diet and drug therapy.

GROUP D (cholesterol 5.2 to 7.8 mmol per litre/triglyceride 2.3 to 5.6 mmol per litre)

CHD risk: high.

Management plan:

i) No other CHD risk factors

Step I: Advise lipid lowering diet and weight reducing diet if appropriate. Correct any underlying causes.
↓
Step II: Re-assess at 2 to 4 months
If treatment goal achieved re-assess at 6 to 12 months. If treatment goal not achieved then check compliance with diet and weight control and check control of underlying causes.
↓
Step III: Re-assess at 3 to 6 months
↓
Step IV: Re-assess at 3 to 6 months
If treatment goal reached, re-assess at one year. If treatment goal not reached then consider drug therapy.

Long term: Re-assess at 1 to 5 yearly intervals if treated by diet alone; and at 3-monthly intervals increasing to one yearly if diet and drugs used. Continue drug therapy only if justified by the response.

ii) Other CHD risk factors present

Step I: as in i) plus control of associated risk factors
↓
Step II: Re-assess at 3 to 6 months
As in i)
↓
Step III: Re-assess at 3 to 6 months
Treatment goal achieved re-assess at one year. If treatment goal not achieved then consider drug therapy.
↓
Step IV: Re-assess at 3 months
If treatment goal achieved, re-assess at one year. If treatment goal not achieved, re-assess drug therapy and diet.

Long term: Re-assess at 1 to 5 yearly intervals if treated by diet alone; and at 3-monthly intervals increasing to one year if treated by diet and drugs. Continue drug therapy only if justified by the response.

GROUP E (cholesterol >7.8 mmol per litre/triglyceride >5.6 mmol per litre)

CHD risk: Some patients in this group will be at very high risk of CHD.

Investigations: Investigate and correct underlying causes. Make precise diagnosis of primary lipid disorder (see Chapter 6) wherever possible. Consider referral to specialist centre for treatment.

Management plan:

Step I: Lipid lowering diet and weight control (except for chylomicronaemia syndrome for which a low-fat diet will be needed). Control any associated risk factors.
↓
Step II: Re-assess at 1 to 3 months
If treatment goal achieved re-assess at 4 to 6 months. If treatment goal not achieved then drug therapy will probably be required. The choice of drug will be dependent on the type of lipid disorder present.
↓
Step III: Re-assess lipid response and side-effects at 1 to 2 months
If treatment goal achieved re-assess at 4 to 6 months. If treatment goal not achieved adjust drug dosage and maximise dietary compliance. Check both that underlying causes are corrected and that any associated CHD risk factors are controlled.
↓
Step IV: Re-assess lipid response and side-effects at 1 to 2 months
As for step III.
↓
Step V: Re-assess at 2 to 4 months
If treatment goal achieved re-assess at one year. If treatment goal still not achieved then adjust dose of drug and/or consider introduction of second drug.

Long term: Re-assess at three-monthly intervals increasing to one year. Continue drugs only if justified by response and assess cardiovascular status at 1 to 5 yearly intervals.

WHICH DRUG?

It is apparent from reading through the above management plan that only rarely are drugs indicated and then only after diet has been tried for many months and the doctor is certain that the patient is using it properly.

The following are some simple guidelines to follow when finally considering drug use.

Group A: Drugs will only very rarely be needed in this group. Non-responders will usually just not be complying properly with the diet.

Group B: Use bile acid sequestrants at low dosages. Nicotinic acid or fibrate or HMG-CoA reductase inhibitor should be considered as second-line therapies.

Group C: Drug treatment is controversial in this group. Consider either nicotinic acid or a fibrate or fish oil.

Group D:

i)   If cholesterol remains elevated, triglyceride within normal limits – use nicotinic acid, or fibrate, or bile acid sequestrant or HMG-CoA reductase inhibitor.

ii)   If cholesterol within normal limits, but triglyceride raised – use fibrate or nicotinic acid.

iii)   Both cholesterol and triglyceride elevated – use fibrate or nicotinic acid or fibrate plus bile acid sequestrant, or HMG-CoA reductase inhibitor.

Group E: Choice of drug depends on type of lipid disorder.

i)   Familial hypercholesterolaemia – bile acid sequestrants or HMG-CoA reductase inhibitor or nicotinic acid. If the response is inadequate use combination therapy – bile acid sequestrants plus either nicotinic acid or fibrate or HMG-CoA reductase inhibitor.

ii)   Remnant hyperlipidaemia – fibrate or nicotinic acid.

iii)   Familial hypertriglyceridaemia –nicotinic acid or fibrate.

iv)   Familial combined hyperlipidaemia – as in Group D.

v)   Primary chylomicronaemia – drug treatment is rarely needed.

FOLLOW UP

It is important that these patients are all followed adequately to ensure compliance with and efficacy of the treatment.

Patients on a lipid lowering diet should be seen after three or four months, then one to four times a year depending on the severity of the problem. On each occasion, fasting lipids should be checked.

Groups A and C – these patients can be seen every two to five years when controlled or every one to two years if any risk factors are present.

Groups B, D and E – these patients are seen about six times a year until control is established. Once controlled they need to be seen only every one to three years (less for those on a diet), and every three months for those taking medication.

A simpler alternative

If the above seems too complicated (and to be honest it can look that way if you don't take time to follow it through) then the Family Heart Association has a more basic classification:

Patient group	1st-line therapy	2nd-line therapy
Hypercholesterolaemia	Resin	Resin and fibrate or HMG-CoA reductase inhibitor
Mixed hyperlipidaemia	Fibrate	HMG-CoA reductase inhibitor or resin + nicotinic acid
Hypertriglyceridaemias	Rarely need ?	Nicotinic acid or fibrate

---

9
Classification of hyperlipidaemias

This chapter contains information on the following:

Part I: Secondary hyperlipidaemias
- Diabetes
- Alcohol abuse
- Medication
- Hypothyroidism
- Renal disease

Part II: Primary hyperlipidaemias
- Common hyperlipidaemia
- Familial hypercholesterolaemia
- Remnant hyperlipidaemia
- Familial combined hyperlipidaemia
- Chylomicronaemia syndrome
- Familial hypertriglyceridaemia
- Primary HDL abnormalities

The classification of hyperlipidaemias has never been one of the most exciting topics in medicine.

In the past the teaching of the subject revolved around the World Health Organisation's 'Fredrickson' classification of primary hyperlipidaemias. This classified lipids on the basis of the electrophoretic patterns and tended to boggle the mind with long lists of arrows showing one or more of the lipoproteins LDL, HDL, VLDL or chylomicrons to be raised or lowered.

In reality there is no need for the classification of this common condition to present too much of a problem. Nor is there any good reason why, once hyperlipidaemia has been diagnosed, some form of more specific diagnosis should not be made.

Certainly it is useful to know exactly which hyperlipidaemia is present since the many different varieties have widely differing prognoses and methods of management. Although of less use when the levels of cholesterol and triglyceride are relatively low, the need to make a proper diagnosis becomes increasingly important as the levels get higher. At the very highest levels, a knowledge of which hyperlipidaemia is present can be vitally important. Thus the GP ignores this classification at his/her peril.

So, to start simply, hyperlipidaemias can be split into primary and secondary. We will look at each in turn.

PART I: SECONDARY HYPERLIPIDAEMIAS

It may seem odd to begin with the causes of secondary hyperlipidaemia, but in purely clinical terms this is the first step in management; therefore it must be appropriate to look at them first.

The most common causes of secondary hyperlipidaemia are:

Diabetes mellitus   Cholestasis
Alcohol abuse   Chronic renal failure
Medications   Nephrotic syndrome
Obesity   Bulimia
Hypothyroidism

Table 6. Some causes of secondary hyperlipidaemia

	Main lipid abnormaility	Lipoprotein changes		
		Chylomicrons	VLDL	LDL	HDL
Diabetes mellitus	↑ triglyceride	↑	↑		↓
Alcohol abuse	↑ triglyceride	↑	↑		
Drugs	↑ triglyceride and/or ↑ cholesterol				
Hypothyroidism	↑ cholesterol			↑	
Chronic renal failure	↑ triglyceride		↑	↑ or N	
Nephrotic syndrome	↑ cholesterol and ↑ triglyceride		↑	↑	
Cholestasis	↑ cholesterol			↑	↓
Bulimia	↑ triglyceride	↑	↑		

These can usually be diagnosed by ensuring you ask appropriate questions when taking the initial history and by clinical examination. A biochemical profile (for glucose, γ-GT, LFTs, urea and creatinine) is a useful first investigation.

If hyperlipidaemia is caused by one of the above then their removal will usually improve the situation (although it should not be forgotten that secondary and primary hyperlipidaemias can exist together).

The risk of CHD is often less marked in secondary hyperlipidaemias since the duration of the problem is usually shorter (with the notable exception of diabetes).

Diabetes

Insulin is an important factor in the normal metabolism of lipids in the body; thus any deficiency can produce an abnormal lipid profile in the bloodstream.

Diabetics show a threefold increase in the incidence of CHD and this is probably largely due to abnormalities in lipid metabolism.

One of the most important roles of insulin is in the catabolism of triglyceride-rich lipoproteins since the hormone is needed for the normal functioning of lipoprotein lipase. Without it, triglyceride levels and to a lesser extent, cholesterol levels become raised (especially in Type II diabetics).

In diabetics with chronic untreated disease, tendon xanthomata may appear, but these will regress once insulin levels are returned to normal with medication.

Generally, lipoprotein levels revert to normal once the hyperglycaemia has been effectively treated. In some NIDDM patients however, usually because of obesity or co-existence of familial hypertriglyceridaemia, the lipoprotein levels do not get back completely to normal.

On top of controlling the blood sugar level, every effort must be made to control the intake of fats and cholesterol. However, since the diabetic diet is almost identical in terms of its fat content, to a lipid lowering diet, the diabetic should already be following the correct dietary guidelines.

Since CHD is so much more likely in these patients, it is worth considering drug treatment earlier if lipid levels are persistently elevated despite good compliance with a diet. A fibrate is the drug of choice.

Alcohol abuse

Although not often something volunteered readily by most patients, alcohol abuse is a relatively common cause of secondary hyperlipidaemia – again mainly hypertriglyceridaemia rather than hypercholesterolaemia.

Alcohol acts in the liver to inhibit fatty acid activation and to increase fatty acid synthesis, thus increasing VLDL production. As little as 15 units a week could be enough to cause a rise in levels in some individuals.

Pancreatitis is a major complication in patients with very high levels of triglyceride.

The hypertriglyceridaemia will often disappear within 14 days of reducing alcohol intake.

Medication

A number of commonly used drugs can cause moderate hyperlipidaemia. These include:

Thiazides and other diuretics
Combined oral contraceptives
Retinoids
Corticosteroids

The effects (usually an elevation in serum cholesterol levels) usually disappear on stopping or swapping the drug.

The effect on lipid levels of the oral contraceptive pill is one of the most well documented.

Oestrogens tend to raise serum triglyceride and HDL levels, while decreasing LDL levels. Progestogens however have exactly the opposite effect. The net effect in some of the older pills was for LDL to rise and HDL to fall, the effects increasing the longer the pill was taken.

It is now judged that there does not seem to be any overall increase in the incidence of CHD in pill-taking women.

Obesity

Obese patients tend to have a relatively poor glucose tolerance; thus like diabetics they tend to have raised levels of triglyceride as well. Weight reduction often reduces the triglyceride problem as well as any excess cholesterol.

Hypothyroidism (Figure 8)

Hypothyroidism may be evident from a history of intolerance to cold, constipation, menorrhagia, hair loss and so on. In these cases a thyroid function test is confirmatory. A family history of thyroid disease is common.

Thyroxine appears to enhance the activity of lipoprotein lipase and that of cell surface lipoprotein receptors thus leading to a rise in LDL and total cholesterol levels. Triglyceride levels may also be raised.

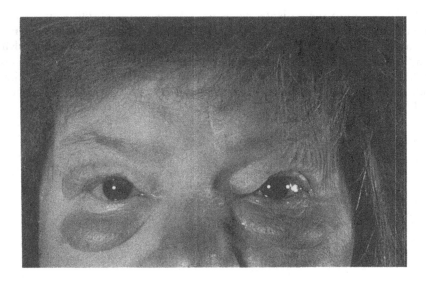

Figure 8. Myxoedematous patients commonly suffer raised cholesterol levels (National Medical Slide Bank)

It is not uncommon to see cholesterol levels in the 9 to 20 mmol per litre range in these patients.

Control of the thyroid disease will lead to a normalisation of lipid levels.

Renal disease

Cardiovascular disease is one of the most common complications seen in patients receiving haemodialysis. Triglyceride and cholesterol levels are raised as a result of interference with hepatic and lipoprotein lipase.

In nephrotic syndrome the exact cause of the often seen hyperlipidaemia is unclear – it may be that the hypoalbuminaemia causes fatty acids to be taken up more easily by the liver, thus increasing VLDL synthesis.

General points

Cholesterol and triglyceride levels should be re-checked about 4 to 6 weeks after the secondary causes have been dealt with.

Since both primary and secondary hyperlipidaemia may exist together it must be remembered that the secondary cause may lead to some modification in the treatments used to treat the raised lipid. Diets in particular should be very carefully tailored to the patient's needs in diabetes and nephrotic syndrome. In these cases it may indeed be best to employ the help of a community dietician.

Similarly, if a patient is being treated with one set of drugs for the underlying condition causing their secondary hyperlipidaemia, then the GP should make sure that there are no interactions or adverse effects that could worsen either condition – for example some fibrates should be given in reduced dosage in renal failure.

PART II: PRIMARY HYPERLIPIDAEMIAS (Table 7)

This may sound rather facile, but if all secondary causes of hyperlipidaemia have been ruled out, then the patient must have some form of primary hyperlipidaemia. The question is, which one?

Pointless though it may at first appear to a busy GP, it is possible to make a precise diagnosis in a large number of cases and, in fact, this can be an extremely useful and important exercise.

Clinical experience has shown that a patient's prognosis can vary quite dramatically depending upon which primary hyperlipidaemia is present. Ignorance of exactly what sort it is can mean that the condition is treated less (or more) vigorously than is warranted and that the patients themselves are inadequately informed of the prognosis. Arriving at a formal diagnosis may mean spending a little more time with the patient than you might otherwise, but time thus spent can pay dividends later.

Complicated additional tests are rarely needed since the diagnosis will usually become obvious from the family history, physical examination and lipid measurements. If special studies are needed then these may be best organised by a specialist centre.

In the future genetic techniques will undoubtedly play an important part in making a diagnosis and indeed they will probably allow more types of hyperlipidaemia to be discerned.

COMMON OR POLYGENIC HYPERLIPIDAEMIA

This is undoubtedly the commonest type of hyperlipidaemia, the diagnosis being made by exclusion of all the other sorts. The great majority of people in the UK with higher than normal serum cholesterol will usually fall into this category having no family history of CHD or hyperlipidaemia and no abnormal physical signs.

The cause of the disease is by no means simple. A number of different genes (as yet we are not sure exactly which) interact with environmental factors such as a high-cholesterol diet and obesity to push up the cholesterol in the blood.

Family history: not particularly helpful, but there may occasionally be a family history of CHD.

Table 7 Classification of primary hyperlipidaemias

Type of hyperlipidaemia	Frederickson lipoprotein phenotype	Typical lipid levels (mmol per litre)	Lipoprotein	CHD risk	Pancreatitis risk	Clinical signs
Polygenic hypercholesterolaemia	IIa	cholesterol: 6.5 to 9.0 triglyceride: <2.3	LDL↑ HDL→↓	+	–	xanthelasma, corneal arcus
Familial combined (mixed) hyperlipidaemia	IIa, IIb or IV	cholesterol: 6.5 to 10.0 triglyceride: 2.5 to 12.0	VLDL↑→ LDL↑→ HDL→↓	+ +	–	corneal arcus, xanthelasma
Familial hypercholesterolaemia	IIa or IIb	cholesterol: 7.5 to 16.0 triglyceride: <5.0	LDL↑ VLDL→↑ HDL→↓	+ + +	–	tendon xanthomata, corneal arcus, xanthelasma
Remnant particle disease (dysbetalipoproteinaemia)	III	cholesterol: 9.0 to 14.0 triglyceride: 9.0 to 14.0	LDL↑ HDL→↓	+ + +	+	pulmar xanthomata occasional tendon xanthomata
Chylomicronaemia syndrome (lipoprotein lipase deficiency, apoprotein C-II deficiency)	I	cholesterol: <6.5 triglyceride: 10.0 to 30.0	chylomicrons ↑	–	+ + +	eruptive xanthomata, lipaemia retinalis, hepatosplenomegaly
Familial hypertriglyceridaemia	IV or V	cholesterol: 6.5 to 12.0 triglyceride: 10.0 to 30.0	VLDL↑ chylomicrons →↑	?	+ +	eruptive xanthomata, lipaemia retinalis, hepatosplenomegaly
HDL abnormalities						
hypoalphalipoproteinaemia	–	HDL cholesterol: <0.9	HDL↓	+ +	–	–
hyperalphalipoproteinaemia	–	HDL cholesterol: >2.0	HDL↑	–	–	–

From *Mims Magazine*

Examination:	Tendon xanthomata never appear. Corneal arcus and xanthelasma may be seen (Figure 9). Sometimes obese.
Lipids:	Cholesterol and LDL increased, but usually only mild to moderate rise. Triglyceride – normal.

CHD risk: moderate.

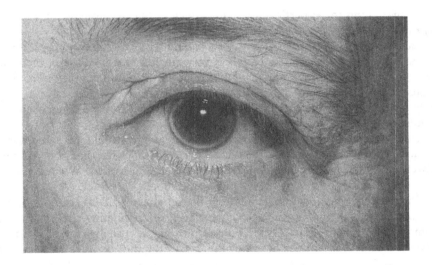

Figure 9. Corneal arcus and xanthelasma – both classical signs of familial hyper-cholesterolaemia (National Medical Slide Bank)

FAMILIAL HYPERCHOLESTEROLAEMIA

Familial hypercholesterolaemia (FH) is now the best understood of the primary hyperlipidaemias. It is also one of the most serious.

The disease is inherited as an autosomal dominant; thus both heterozygous and homozygous forms of the disease exist (Figure 10).

The heterozygous form affects about one in 500 people making it one of the commonest major genetic disorders in the world. Lebanese and South African

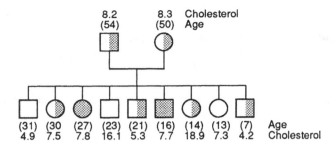

Figure 10. The pedigree of a Lebanese family, showing the inheritance of FH. Unshaded individuals are unaffected, half-shaded are heterozygous and shaded are homozygous.

Afrikaaners tend to be particularly badly affected, but the disease can occur in any race.

The average GP will have at least one patient with familial hypercholesterolaemia in their practice, and since this is very much a 'family' disease, there are likely to be a lot more if the patient's relatives also live in the area. It is estimated that there are about 100,000 cases in the UK, yet only a small proportion, probably less than 20 per cent have so far been diagnosed and treated.

Men who inherit the heterozygous form have an 8 to 10-fold increased risk of developing CHD and if left untreated, 85 per cent will have had a myocardial infarct and about half of them will have died by the age of 60. Women tend to have a better prognosis, CHD developing some 10–15 years later.

The underlying defect is a decrease in the number of LDL receptors on the cell surfaces and this means that the level of circulating LDL can rise dramatically (Figure 11). Hypercholesterolaemia is usually severe, usually between 9 and 12 mmol per litre, but values of 7.8 mmol per litre and above in adults and 6.7 mmol per litre and above in children are compatible with the diagnosis. The condition can in fact be diagnosed at birth from umbilical cord blood (although this is not generally felt to be particularly accurate).

Triglyceride levels are normal or slightly elevated.

The characteristic physical signs of familial hypercholesterolaemia are tendon xanthomata. These are sometimes difficult to spot and should therefore be looked for specifically on the Achilles tendons and on the extensor tendons of the hand and more rarely at the insertion of the patellar tendons. These patients will also usually have xanthelasma and corneal arcus, but these occur frequently in other types of hyperlipidaemia and thus are not pathognomonic for the condition.

Although characteristic of the disease and a great help in diagnosis, xanthomata are not always present, particularly in the younger family members;

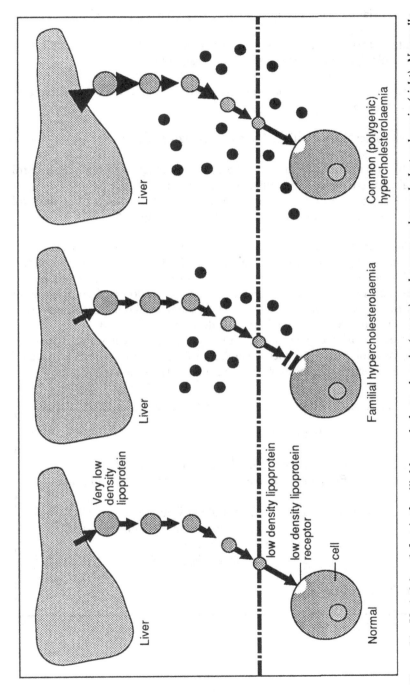

Figure 11. *Underlying defect in familial hypercholesterolaemia (centre) and common hypercholesterolaemia (right). Normally, a receptor recognises LDL-cholesterol and removes it from the circulation. In familial hypercholesterolaemia, there is a defect in this receptor, leading to raised LDL levels. In common hypercholesterolaemia, the receptor is usually normal, but too much LDL-cholesterol is produced*

thus other criteria for diagnosis must be looked for. These include:

- a definite history in a first-degree relative (parent, brother, sister or children) of myocardial infarction occuring before the age of 60.

- a definite history in a second-degree relative of a myocardial infarction before the age of 50.

- a cholesterol level greater than 7.8 in a first-degree relative.

A combination of one or more of the above together with high cholesterol levels (as above) are enough to confirm the diagnosis.

Diet alone is not usually sufficient to bring down their levels of cholesterol sufficiently, thus drug therapy is usually needed (see Chapter 5).

The homozygous form is much more rare affecting only one person per million in most countries. Here the cell surface LDL receptors are completely absent and as a result the levels of plasma cholesterol are astronomically high – usually between 15 and 25 mmol per litre. Patients develop rapidly progressive CHD and rarely live beyond the age of 30. Tendon xanthomata, corneal arcus and aortic stenosis, even frank CHD usually develop in childhood.

Even after intensive treatment, which these days can include ileal bypassing and even plasmaphoresis (a process similar to renal dialysis where a machine filters out all the excess cholesterol from the blood), the prognosis is poor.

Family history: Definite (as above).

Examination: Tendon xanthomata diagnostic (Figure 12)
                      Frequent xanthelasma corneal arcus before 40 years.

Lipids: Cholesterol   >7.8 mmol per litre
                                   >6.7 mmol per litre (under age of 16)
                LDL Cholesterol > 4.9 mmol per litre
                Triglyceride – normal or slightly raised.

CHD risk: Very high.

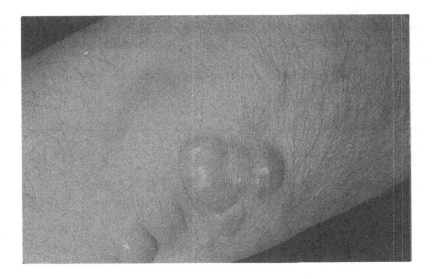

Figure 12. Tuberous tendon xanthomata – pathognomonic of remnant hyper-lipidaemia (National Medical Slide Bank)

REMNANT HYPERLIPIDAEMIA

This is a much rarer condition than familial hypercholesterolaemia; the frequency of the disease is only about one in 5000; nevertheless it is an important cause of early onset of CHD, peripheral vascular disease and cerebrovascular disease.

The underlying lipid abnormality is rather complex, but essentially there is a rise in both cholesterol and triglyceride caused by an accumulation of cholesterol-rich VLDL.

Ultracentrifugation of the VLDL reveals that the ratio of cholesterol to triglyceride is 0.6 or above, this increase in cholesterol being due to the accumulation of remnant particles from the hydrolysis of chylomicrons and VLDL by lipoprotein lipase.

Normally these particles are removed in the liver, but in patients with this condition there is a genetic defect in the apolipoprotein (apo E3) that normally recognises it. This defect, combined with the presence of other inherited hyperlipidaemias and secondary causes such as diabetes, renal disease or hypothyroidism will lead to the condition developing.

In practice the condition is usually diagnosed by the presence of almost pathognomonic orange/yellow streaks in the palmar creases (planar xanthomata) and eruptive soft tissue xanthomata (tuberous xanthomata) on the elbows and knees.

Although the condition can be diagnosed in childhood, it is not usually evident until later in life. CHD will often develop in the 40s and 50s, but in a young lean individual a moderate hypertriglyceridaemia may be the only manifestation.

Obesity, glucose intolerance and hyperuricaemia are all frequently associated with the condition.

Family history:	not always obvious
Examination:	palmar xanthomata (in 50 per cent of cases) tuberous xanthomata on elbows and knees
Lipids:	cholesterol ↑ triglyceride ↑
CHD risk:	very high

FAMILIAL COMBINED HYPERLIPIDAEMIA

This is a rather confusing condition. The patient may have both raised cholesterol and triglyceride levels; alternatively they may have pure hyper-cholesterolaemia or hypertriglyceridaemia. These lipid patterns may change with time – often on repeat testing the lipids will be quite different, particularly with regard to the triglycerides.

Patients do not tend to have xanthomata and in general the level of lipid in their blood is only moderately raised. Nevertheless, there is always a very strong family history of CHD (the condition appearing in every generation) and a high incidence of CHD in the individuals concerned. Typically, the pattern of hyperlipidaemia varies throughout the family.

Thus familial combined hyperlipidaemia should be suspected in any individual with mild hyperlipidaemia but a personal or strong family history of CHD.

The underlying problem is obviously a genetic one, probably autosomal dominant, with a prevalence as high as one in 300 (making it the most common inherited primary hyperlipidaemia). There is an overproduction of apolipo-protein B, the building protein of VLDL and LDL and thus either or both these lipoproteins are increased depending upon the efficiency of the lipoprotein catabolism in that patient.

Family history:	very strong history of CHD in every generation pattern of hyperlipidaemia varies among family members
Examination:	no xanthomata
Lipids:	both cholesterol and triglyceride ↑ (only mild to moderate) or cholesterol ↑ or triglyceride ↑
CHD risk:	high

CHYLOMICRONAEMIA SYNDROME (Figure 13)

This is a mixture of a number of rare conditions all leading to the accumulation of chylomicrons in the blood stream and severe hypertriglyceridaemia. These patients typically have crops of eruptive xanthomata and/or recurrent episodes of acute pancreatitis. The risk of CHD is not high.

The condition is caused by a deficiency of the enzyme lipoprotein lipase or of the apolipoprotein C2 which activates it. The inheritance is autosomal recessive.

The precise diagnosis can only be arrived at in hospital. A positive fat-deprivation test, in which the patient has a fat-free diet for three days, is shown by an 80 per cent reduction in plasma triglyceride and virtual disappearance of chylomicronaemia. Levels of apo-C2 and lipoprotein lipase can then be assayed in specialist centres.

Clinically these patients have eruptive xanthomata and heptosplenomegaly due to the accumulation of fat-laden macrophages. The chylomicrons also tend to plug the capillaries in the pancreas leading to pancreatitis. Unfortunately in this condition, the levels of plasma amylase are not a reliable measure of whether pancreatitis is present or not; thus any abdominal pain should be investigated by measuring the urinary amylase/creatinine ratio.

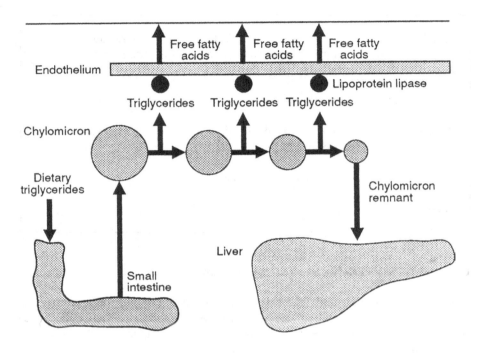

Figure 13. Metabolism of chylomicrons. Chylomicrons transport dietary triglyceride (TG) into the circulation. TG is hydrolysed by lipoprotein lipase to free fatty acids which are taken up by the tissues. The liver removes chlyomicron remnants

Family history:	unusual.
Physical examination:	eruptive xanthomata, hepatosplenomegaly, retinal lipaemia.
Lipids:	cholesterol ↑ (mild to moderate) triglyceride >10 mmol per litre (fasting), but may reach as high as 100 mmol per litre.
CHD risk:	low.
Pancreatitis risk:	very high

FAMILIAL HYPERTRIGLYCERIDAEMIA

This is a similar condition to chylomicronaemia syndrome, except the lipoprotein lipase and apo-C2 levels are unchanged. The underlying metabolic derangement is unknown.

These patients have moderate to very high levels of plasma triglyceride due to an overproduction of VLDL (sometimes chylomicronaemia is also present).

Diagnosis is made both by studying the family history which will show an autosomal dominant transmission, and by performing the fat-deprivation test which exagerates rather than ameliorates the condition. The disorder rarely manifests itself before adult life and may present with pancreatitis.

There is an association with venous thrombosis and diabetis mellitus.

Family history:	strong
Physical examination:	eruptive xanthomata lipaemia retinalis hepatosplenomegaly
Lipids:	cholesterol ↑ (mild to moderate) triglyceride ↑ (but not usually as high as chylomicronaemia syndrome)
CHD risk:	low
Pancreatitis risk:	high

PRIMARY HDL ABNORMALITIES

Occasionally mild hypercholesterolaemia can be caused by a high level of HDL. This is a benign condition (the so-called longevity syndrome since it is associated with increased life expectancy), seen particularly in post-menopausal women on hormone replacement therapy, in patients on enzyme-inducing drugs such as phenytoin and phenobarbitone, and sometimes it is familial.

In contrast, low HDL levels which are sometimes found in association with an apolipoprotein A1 gene deficiency affects about 4 per cent of the population. This condition is associated with an increased incidence of CHD.

10
Costs and benefits

This chapter contains information on the following:

- Cost of cholesterol testing
- Cost of treating hyperlipidaemia
- Cost of drugs
- Cost of diet
- Cost–benefit

No discussion of cholesterol screening and the prevention of CHD can be complete without looking at the costs involved and the benefits that might accrue. Happily much of this information has recently been provided by the Department of Health Standing Medical Advisory Committee (SMAC) in its recently published report on 'The cost effectiveness of opportunistic cholesterol testing'.

I make no apology for repeating much of their work since it is certainly the most up-to-date available.

THE COST OF TESTING FOR HYPERLIPIDAEMIA

First let's look at the precise costs involved in actually testing a patient for his or her cholesterol level. The SMAC estimated that if tested using a hospital analyser, laboratory costs for each test would be on average 65p per sample. This assumes that half of all tests are for blood cholesterol alone and half for cholesterol, HDL, and triglyceride. And it includes the cost of more detailed tests for about 12,000 patients each year who are found to have severe hyperlipidaemia.

Extra costs include the cost of syringe needle and vial – 18p, and the cost of professional time to take it – £2.00. The total cost would therefore be about £2.80.

THE COST OF TREATING HYPERLIPIDAEMIA

Obviously the cost of treating hyperlipidaemia varies according to which guide to clinical practice is followed (European Atherosclerosis Society/British Hyperlipidaemia Association/US National Cholesterol Education Programme and so on).

Costings are assumed based on the following regimen:

Table 8. Testing and treatment over 10 years

Blood cholesterol	No. of tests	No. of 20 minute counselling sessions
<5.2	1	1
5.2 – 6.5		
non-smokers	2	2
smokers	4	4
6.5 – 7.8	7	7
>7.8	15	15

Counselling

The first step taken in each case is to provide counselling. Every patient tested will obviously require some form of counselling and this may be provided by either the GP or, more frequently with the advent of the new contract, the practice nurse. It is estimated that a GP costs between £25 and £45 per hour and a practice nurse £6 per hour. A final costing of £9 per hour for an average session assumes that the practice nurse will shoulder most of the work.

Diet

To some extent the cost of diet as a treatment is essentially zero since the State itself is not directly providing the food that the patient will eat. A campaign to encourage healthy eating and the reduction of risk factors such as smoking and obesity would have a price however. The government recently announced it was about to launch just such a campaign through the Health Education Authority. They have earmarked £25 million for it.

Drugs

The proportion of patients who could eventually be prescribed lipid-lowering agents is uncertain. It can be estimated, using lipid clinic data, that between 4 and 5 per cent will eventually need them, but of course it should be remembered that these are the most 'difficult' patients. A more accurate 'national' figure can only be arrived at by reviewing GP prescribing of these drugs. A telephone survey revealed that only between 1 and 2 per cent of patients with hyperlipidaemia seen in general practice are given drugs.

Naturally the cost of drug treatment depends on which drugs are prescribed. Cholestyramine is the most popular first choice in the UK at present. A dose of 4 sachets a day (that needed for severe cases) costs approximately £600 per patient per year. It's patent runs out however in November 1990 and the costs may fall.

A less expensive drug, bezafibrate for example, will cost only about £110 per year, with the HMG-CoA reductase inhibitor, simvastatin lying roughly in between (a 10 or 20 mg a day dose costing £240 and £405 per year, respectively). More expensive still, obviously, would be a combination of therapies.

Benefits

The likely benefit of blood cholesterol reduction has been estimated for a number of patient groups. Obviously in order to assess any benefit the relative risk to the patient must also be worked out. Based on MRFIT data the following risk ratios were calculated based on the idea that the population's average risk of developing CHD was 1.

Blood cholesterol	Risk ratio
<6.5	0.65
⩾6.5	
diet only	1.52
drug treatment in	
more severe hyperlipidaemia,	
i.e. >8.0	4.00

Each CHD death prevented in middle age causes an average gain in life expectancy of 17 years. There is also a gain associated with the avoidance of a non-fatal heart attack.

A successful intervention programme will therefore reduce the costs of NHS treatment. The Office of Health Education suggests a cost of £2800 per patient ultimately dying of CHD.

The SMAC estimated that, should a national coronary risk factor reduction programme be introduced, then a likely cholesterol level reduction of 5% in those with a cholesterol level of <6.5 mmol/L and 15% in those >6.5 mmol/L, would lead to an annual saving of almost 8000 lives at a total cost per annum of £271 million.

However these estimates assume a high rate of drug prescribing since they are based on the experience of hospital lipid clinics. Since GPs prescribe less often, the total cost could be half or even a quarter of the above.

These estimates therefore suggest that a testing programme, however it is introduced, could be associated with a major reduction in mortality, particularly among middle-aged men in whom there are about 50,000 CHD deaths each year in England and Wales.

In comparison it has been estimated that the cervical cancer screening programme may save only 1000 lives per year and the breast cancer screening programme only a few hundred. The cost–benefit for some sort of intervention in this area is thus extremely favourable.

Overall, then, a programme of testing high-risk groups in general practice, counselling them on diet and lifestyle and if necessary starting them on drugs, makes sense both clinically and economically. Unfortunately the government has not yet given its full backing to a national scheme, but as individuals, GPs have an unparalleled chance to really do something about the morbidity and mortality that exists in their practices.

Appendix I: Lipid metabolism

WHAT ARE LIPIDS?

The word 'lipid' is used to describe a very heterogeneous group of substances each of which are linked together by two facts: that they contain one or more fatty acid and that they are insoluble in water.

Fatty acids are long-chain molecules made up of carbon, hydrogen and oxygen atoms. They are usually classified as being either saturated, meaning all the possible carbon bonds are linked to a hydrogen bond, or unsaturated, meaning that there are a number of unlinked carbon bonds, necessitating the formation of a double bond. Fatty acids with more than one double bond are thus polyunsaturated.

Most animal fats such as stearic acid are saturated, while most vegetable fats (e.g. linoleic acid) and many marine fats, such as eicosapentaenoic acid are polyunsaturated. Olive oil contains mainly oleic acid, a monounsaturated fatty acid.

The lipids that circulate in human plasma are naturally made up (to varying degrees) of fatty acids. Obviously the ultimate source of these fatty acids is the diet.

Plasma lipids include cholesterol (70 per cent of which is esterified with a fatty acid), triglyceride, phospholipids and free fatty acids.

Cholesterol: Cholesterol exists both in esterified an unesterified forms. Biochemically it is a precursor of bile acids, all steroid hormones and vitamin D. It is also a major component of all cell membranes.

The body has two sources of cholesterol:

1) the body itself through catabolism
2) diet – meat, fish, poultry, egg yolks and dairy products.

Triglycerides: These are a major source of energy for the body. Most of the body's triglyceride is obtained in the diet, but it can also be produced by the body itself.

Triglycerides make up about 95 per cent of the lipid content of adipose tissue.

Phospholipids are major components of cell walls.

Free fatty acids circulate both intra- and extracellularly taking part in various metabolic processes to produce energy. When in the blood stream they are bound to serum albumin.

PUT SIMPLY, HOW ARE LIPIDS METABOLISED IN THE BODY?

Let's start from the point where fats are ingested in our diet and work through to their final utilisation at a cellular level (Figure 14).

First, it is important to remember that fats are an important energy source and that they are present naturally in an awful lot of the foods we eat. The normal Western diet contains about 40 per cent fat.

Unfortunately fats are insoluble in their natural state; thus, to get over this, the body has had to provide a complex system for absorbing them and then transporting them around the body.

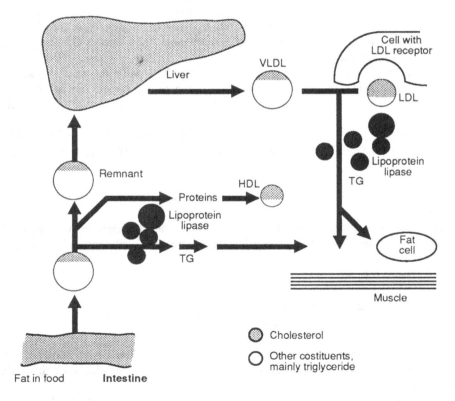

Figure 14. Simplified outline of lipoprotein metabolism

1. Absorption of fat in the diet

Fats in the gut lumen are partially hydrolysed by enzymes (lipases) secreted by glands in the small intestinal villi and then formed into micelles (tiny globules of hydrolysed fat) with the help of bile acids secreted by the liver.

Non-esterified fatty acids and monoglycerides can now be absorbed by the epithelial cells in the duodenum and proximal jejunum and immediately re-esterified into triglycerides. Dietary cholesterol is hydrolysed by pancreatic enzymes and then absorbed, again by the small intestine.

Once through the barrier of the intestinal epithelial cells, this soup of insoluble triglycerides, cholesterol and so on must now be transported to other parts of the body. The body does this by combining cholesterol (both free and esterified), triglyceride, phospholipids and proteins (called apolipoproteins) together in the intestinal wall to form a 'lipoprotein'.

Lipoproteins can be thought of as 'taxis' that deliver lipids to the various parts of the body.

There are five different types of lipoprotein (Figure 15):

VLDL (very low density lipoprotein)
LDL   (low density lipoprotein)
HDL   (high density lipoprotein)
IDL   (intermediate density lipoprotein)
Chylomicrons

2. Chylomicrons and VLDL

The first lipoproteins to be formed are the chylomicrons. These triglyceride-rich complexes are initially secreted into the intestinal lymphatic system, then transported up to the thoracic duct and into the blood stream. The chylomicrons' major function is to deliver dietary triglyceride to the tissues.

An enzyme called lipoprotein lipase is present in the endothelium of capillaries supplying a number of tissues, principally the muscles and adipose tissue. This enzyme 'recognises' an apolipoprotein in the chylomicron, hydrolysing the triglyceride to fatty acids that can be absorbed by the tissues themselves to produce energy. Eventually the chylomicrons become totally depleted of triglyceride and only their 'remnants' remain. These remnants are mainly taken up by the liver.

Chylomicrons only appear after a meal and disappear in the fasting state (they have a halflife of only a few minutes).

The other major carrier of triglyceride, even when triglyceride from the diet is not available, is VLDL. VLDL is secreted by the liver, its triglyceride coming mainly from free fatty acids in the blood stream rather than from the diet. Its triglyceride is removed in the tissues by lipoprotein lipase in exactly the same fashion as it occurs with the chylomicrons.

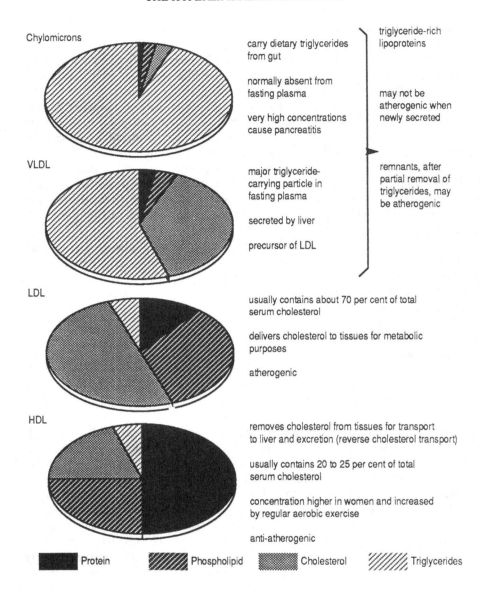

Chylomicrons

carry dietary triglycerides from gut

normally absent from fasting plasma

very high concentrations cause pancreatitis

VLDL

major triglyceride-carrying particle in fasting plasma

secreted by liver

precursor of LDL

LDL

usually contains about 70 per cent of total serum cholesterol

delivers cholesterol to tissues for metabolic purposes

atherogenic

HDL

removes cholesterol from tissues for transport to liver and excretion (reverse cholesterol transport)

usually contains 20 to 25 per cent of total serum cholesterol

concentration higher in women and increased by regular aerobic exercise

anti-atherogenic

triglyceride-rich lipoproteins

may not be atherogenic when newly secreted

remnants, after partial removal of triglycerides, may be atherogenic

Protein   Phospholipid   Cholesterol   Triglycerides

Figure 15. Lipids and lipoproteins. Lipoproteins consist of different mixtures of triglycerides, phospholipids, cholesterol and protein. The greater the proportion of protein present, the higher the density of the particle

3. LDL

The remnants of VLDL are called intermediate density lipoprotein (IDL). Normally some of the IDL is removed by the liver, but most of it is modified further to give rise to low density lipoprotein (LDL).

LDL is the major source of cholesterol for the tissues. Normally about 70 per cent of the total serum content is carried in this form. It circulates in the blood stream, binding with specific LDL receptors on the cell surfaces of many tissues. Once bound by the receptor the LDL is enveloped by the cell and its cholesterol digested in an intracellular lysosome. The LDL-receptor pathway accounts for about two thirds of the LDL catabolised. The rest is catabolised by other LDL receptors in the liver.

4. HDL

High density lipoprotein (HDL) is involved in transporting cholesterol back from the tissues to the liver for excretion. High levels of HDL are thus protective against the development of CHD through the accumulation of too much cholesterol (see below).

Specific sub-types of HDL (HDL3) are secreted both by the liver and by the small intestine. As triglycerides are lost from VLDL and chylomicrons, other constituents are also lost – cholesterol, phospholipid and proteins; these together with cholesterol from the tissues lead to the production of large HDL2 molecules that are then taken up by the liver and excreted. The level of HDL2 in the body is inversely related to the risk of CHD – the more HDL2 the less likely you are to get CHD.

HOW CAN THE PRESENCE OF TOO MUCH FAT AND CHOLESTEROL IN THE DIET CAUSE CHD?

The way the body regulates the amount of cholesterol and other lipids in the body is very complex and for the most part not fully understood.

Certainly the level of cholesterol found in the blood is directly linked to the amount of both cholesterol and saturated fats that are ingested in the diet, but other factors are also involved. These include:
- the amount of cholesterol absorbed in the intestine
- the amount of cholesterol synthesized in the body
- the balance between transportation of cholesterol to the tissues as LDL and then from the tissues as HDL
- the rate of uptake of cholesterol by the tissues
- the amount of cholesterol stored rather than used up by the tissues
- the amount of cholesterol excreted in the bile.

It is certain that the activity of lipoprotein lipase and of the LDL receptors can be regulated to increase or decrease the level of circulating LDL, but exactly how is again not known.

The fact that some people can eat a great deal of fat in their diet and do not have high levels of cholesterol in their blood stream while others eat only a little and do, suggests that certain genetic factors must also be at work. Much research is going on at present to establish what these genetic factors are. Be that as it may, it has been established that in many people the level of cholesterol is higher than is optimal for the body's physiological processes. These individuals thus have to store the cholesterol somewhere or excrete it. Those that cannot excrete enough and thus have continually raised levels of cholesterol in the blood (principally as LDL) have an increased risk of CHD.

The reasons for linking cholesterol with CHD come not only from population studies (see Chapter 2), but also from experimental evidence showing that dietary cholesterol is a major constituent of atherosclerotic plaques (it makes up about one third of its weight). Atherosclerosis is a major cause of CHD.

HOW DOES CHOLESTEROL HELP FORM AN ATHEROSCLEROTIC PLAQUE?

Again the precise mechanism is not clear since plaque formation is a very slow process and may in some circumstances start in early childhood. A brief overview of the present state of knowledge is presented here (Figure 16).

The first event in the process of plaque formation in any vessel seems to be endothelial damage of some kind. The damage may be structural or functional. How this occurs is not known, but it seems likely that factors such as hypertension, cigarette smoking and hypercholesterolaemia are all important in this regard. The net effect however is to allow a greater migration of lipoproteins, principally LDL, in between the cells and into the vessel's intima.

For some reason, which may be linked to the oxidation of LDL in the intima and/or to the presence of abnormal apolipoprotein B (the major apolipoprotein in LDL as well as VLDL and IDL), monocytes are attracted to the damaged endothelial cell surface and they too migrate into the intima, transforming into macrophages and enveloping the LDL.

Over a period of time the macrophages digest more and more LDL until they become bloated with cholesterol. At this point they are known as 'foam cells'. Masses of these cells congregate together in the subendothelial space forming a 'fatty streak'.

Now there is some debate as to whether fatty streaks are in fact the precursors of true atherosclerotic plaques. Fatty streaks can be found in about 45 per cent of infants at autopsy, and they seem just as common in countries which have high levels of CHD as low levels. Nevertheless, it does seem more than likely that at least a proportion of them go on to full-blown plaque formation.

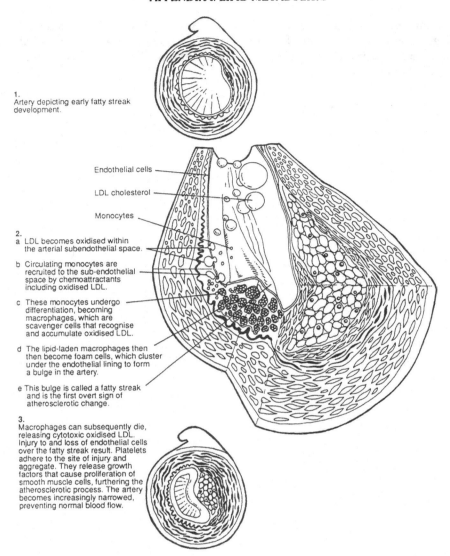

1.
Artery depicting early fatty streak development.

Endothelial cells

LDL cholesterol

Monocytes

2.
a LDL becomes oxidised within the arterial subendothelial space.

b Circulating monocytes are recruited to the sub-endothelial space by chemoattractants including oxidised LDL.

c These monocytes undergo differentiation, becoming macrophages, which are scavenger cells that recognise and accumulate oxidised LDL.

d The lipid-laden macrophages then then become foam cells, which cluster under the endothelial lining to form a bulge in the artery.

e This bulge is called a fatty streak and is the first overt sign of atherosclerotic change.

3.
Macrophages can subsequently die, releasing cytotoxic oxidised LDL. Injury to and loss of endothelial cells over the fatty streak result. Platelets adhere to the site of injury and aggregate. They release growth factors that cause proliferation of smooth muscle cells, furthering the atherosclerotic process. The artery becomes increasingly narrowed, preventing normal blood flow.

Figure 16. The atherosclerotic process

Research suggests that growth factors produced both by the macrophages, endothelial cells and platelets, attract muscle cells and encourage smooth muscle proliferation around the site of the fatty streak.

As the macrophages die, they spill out their enzyme contents, leading to cell necrosis and the attraction of more macrophages. Eventually the typical fibrous plaque, filled with cholesterol and necrotic cells, is formed. This juts out into the vessel lumen causing narrowing and increasing the likelihood of epithelial damage, atherosclerotic fissure formation, platelet aggregation and the eventual development of a thrombus. In this way atherosclerosis directly predisposes to myocardial infarction.

Appendix II: Summary of major trial results

TRIALS OF DIET

Cumulative data from the 10 trials that have been performed so far on the effect of diet on hypercholesterolaemia, show that for a 10 per cent reduction in cholesterol there is a fall of about 13 per cent in the incidence of all coronary heart disease.

Unfortunately a number of these trials were quite small and the majority were carried out in patients who already had CHD.

TRIALS CONTROLLING OTHER RISK FACTORS AND DIET

i) European collaborative trial. Similar-sized factories were chosen in pairs throughout Europe, one being given health education advice, the other acting as a control.

Overall the reduction of CHD was disappointing (only 7.4 per cent), but where risk-factor modification (such as hypertension) had been really successful, the fall in CHD incidence was much more marked.

ii) Oslo study. Men who were at high risk of CHD in that they either smoked and/or they had cholesterol levels of between 7.5 and 9.8 mmol per litre, were split into two groups.

One group had intensive counselling on lipid-lowering diet and stopping smoking, the other acted as a control group.

Over a five-year period the active group showed a 13 per cent fall in cholesterol and big reduction in tobacco consumption. In this group only 31 in 1000 had a coronary event compared with 57 in the control group. Overall mortality was also reduced.

iii) American Multiple Risk Factor Intervention Trial (MRFIT). This massive trial failed to show any great differences between the control and intervention groups, possibly because of the high level of public health advice now being directed to all Americans. The difference in cholesterol levels between the two groups was only 3 per cent.

TRIALS OF LIPID-LOWERING DRUGS AND DIET

Aggregated results from the major drug trials that have been carried out, again show that a 10 per cent reduction in cholesterol will be accompanied by a highly significant reduction of 16 per cent in the incidence of CHD.

i)   World Health Organisation trial of clofibrate. This study showed an impressive reduction in CHD in those taking the drug compared with those who did not. There was a 9 per cent reduction in cholesterol levels.

Unfortunately there was an increased risk of gallstones, together with an increase in all-cause mortality (including cancer deaths and violent deaths) which could not easily be explained. An earlier large trial (the Coronary Drug Project) that also looked at clofibrate did not show this increase in cancer deaths.

ii) The Lipid Research Clinics coronary primary prevention trial of cholestyramine. This studied almost 4000 men who had primary hyper-cholesterolaemia but who had not responded to dietary management.

In the treated group there was a 24 per cent reduction in fatal CHD and a 19 per cent reduction in non-fatal MI. Many of those participating dropped out of the trial during its course, but of those who stuck it out to the end, there was a 39 per cent reduction in all CHD events.

Again, like the WHO trial, there was no reduction in the overall mortality, and there was a slight, but non-significant increase in violent deaths and accidents.

iii) Helsinki Heart Study of gemfibrazil. This study supported the results of the previous two. Four thousand asymptomatic men with LDL plus VLDL above 5.2 mmol per litre were given a lipid-lowering diet and then randomised to either a gemfibrazil or placebo group.

The total number of definite cardiac events was 27 per 1000 in the gemfibrazil group and 41 per 1000 in the placebo group, the non-fatal MI group being affected most (22 against 35 per 1000). These results became apparent after only three years of the trial.

The total mortality was again the same in the two groups; however it must be said that the trial had not set out to investigate this and thus did not have the statistical power to do so. And again there was a slight increase in violent deaths and accidents in the treated group.

Appendix III: Useful addresses

Action on Smoking and Health
5–11 Mortimer Street
London W1N 7RH
Telephone: 071-637-9843

Anticipatory Care Team
The Oxford Centre for Primary Care
Radcliffe Infirmary
Woodstock Road
Oxford, OX2 6HE
Telephone: 0865-817541

British Diabetic Association
10 Queen Anne Street
London, W1M 0BD
Telephone: 071-323-1531

British Heart Foundation
102 Gloucester Place
London, W1H 4DH
Telephone: 071-935-0185

Chest Heart & Stroke Association
Tavistock House North
Tavistock Square
London, WC1H 9JE
Telephone: 071-387-3012

Coronary Prevention Group
60 Great Ormond Street
London, WC1N 3HR
Telephone: 071-833-3687

Diabetes Foundation
177A Tennison Road
London, SE25 5N
Telephone: 081-656-5467

Family Heart Association
9 West Way
Botley
Oxford, OX2 0JB
Telephone: 0865-798969

Heart and Stroke Prevention and
Primary Care
c/o Dr G H Fowler
Department of Community Medicine
and General Practice
Radcliffe Infirmary
Woodstock Road
Oxford, OX2 6HE
Telephone: 0865-511293

Scottish Heart and Arterial Disease
Risk Prevention
c/o Dr M S R McEwan
Faculty of Medicine and Dentistry
Level 10
Ninewells Hospital
Dundee, DD1 9SY
Telephone: 0382-632763, ext. 2763

Index